Praise for
Into the Abyss

'A highly eloquent, fascinating and deeply compassionate book about the continuing mystery of mental illness and the cruel fallacy of seeing it as somehow less real and deserving than so-called physical illness.'

**Henry Marsh CBE, neurosurgeon and
author of *Do No Harm***

'I was expecting this to make my brain hurt, but I was immediately hooked on it… A witty, humane and fascinating book.'

Jo Brand

'Some years ago I told the BMJ that the three biggest influences on me were Anthony Clare, Anthony Soprano and Anthony David. The first sadly is no longer with us, the second never existed, but I am delighted to say that the third has just produced the book we knew he alone could. It's a classic – warm, erudite, and endlessly fascinating. It reminds me of Oliver Sacks in his prime, and there is no higher praise.'

**Sir Simon Wessely, Professor of Psychological
Medicine at King's College London**

'Anthony David brings alive the specialist language of neuropsychiatry – the medical domain where the brain meets the mind – in a series of erudite, insightful and sympathetic accounts of individual patients and their families. This book is written on the basis of a lifetime's clinical experience but readable by anyone who wants to know more about some of the most challenging and perplexing disorders of consciousness, thought and emotion.'

Dr Edward Bullmore, Professor of Psychiatry at the University of Cambridge

'What an insightful and heartfelt book. Professor David's seven in-depth cases expose both the rifts and junctures of the brain and the disordered mind. By emphasizing the subjective inner life of his patients, he provides a welcome antidote to the reductionist thinking of modern medicine while still adhering to sound principles of neuroscience.'

Dr Alan Ropper, Professor of Neurology at Harvard Medical School and author of *Reaching Down the Rabbit Hole: Extraordinary Journeys into the Human Brain*

'Few are better suited to tell the story of our mental lives than Anthony David. He has written a beautiful, intimate book of the stories he's seen, one that probes at the nexus of the biological and societal, of kindness and analysis, of objectivity and empathy, of the individual mind and the social forces that shape it. In his shoes, we get to step into the private realm of the psychiatrist's office, and often into the lingering questions left in the psychiatrist's mind.'

Dr David Eagleman, neuroscientist at Stanford University, internationally bestselling author, creator and host of *The Brain*

'This powerful book can help everyone understand our minds better.'

Dr Rahul Jandial, author of *Life Lessons from a Brain Surgeon*

Into the Abyss

A Neuropsychiatrist's Notes on Troubled Minds

ANTHONY DAVID

ONEWORLD

A Oneworld Book

First published by Oneworld Publications in 2020

ISBN 978-1-78607-705-9 (hardback)
ISBN 978-1-78607-854-4 (export paperback)
eISBN 978-1-78607-706-6

Typeset by Geethik Technologies
Printed and bound in Great Britain by Clays Ltd, Elcograf S.p.A.

Oneworld Publications
10 Bloomsbury Street, London, WC1B 3SR, England
3754 Pleasant Ave, Suite 100, Minneapolis, MN 55409, USA

Stay up to date with the latest books,
special offers, and exclusive content from
Oneworld with our newsletter

Sign up on our website
oneworld-publications.com

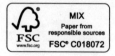

MIX
Paper from
responsible sources
FSC® C018072

For my family

Contents

Introduction

Open a newspaper on any day of the week and there will be an article on mental health or more pertinently, ill-health. We read that the issue is affecting more and more people: the young, the old, women, men. Behaviour we used to take for granted now attracts a diagnosis; we and our families are all on pills or in therapy. Opinion pieces either lament the over-diagnosis and the medicalisation of life, or blame it all on modern society. The real problem, they say, is social media, sexual abuse, drugs, poverty, wealth, patriarchy, feminism, religion, lack of religion…the list goes on.

Stepping back from this cacophony, as a person whose job it is to understand such phenomena, a couple of things strike me. While many of these arguments are plausible, they all tend to take a social or political perspective. By contrast, when people talk to their closest friends about troubles in their lives, the natural tendency is to look only at personal experiences, family problems and relationships. Less commonly, in my experience, do people think about physical illness, biochemical processes, genetics or the brain.

Modern psychiatry weaves together all of these strands – biology, psychology and sociology – to create the 'biopsychosocial' model of mental disorder.[1] We are proud to do so. It shows both our breadth of expertise and rejection of dogma. But applying this model is challenging. Every time we meet a new patient, we must decide which of the three, if any, is most important; otherwise, we are left with a theory that explains everything and nothing.

One way to separate the contribution of genes from the influence of our environment is to study twins who share the same DNA. At the other end of the spectrum, on whole groups of individuals we can look at the effects of war, recession, legalisation of drugs or new treatments. Then there is the more archetypically 'scientific' work carried out in labs: animal experiments or research using brain scanners and other new technologies. But even when such work is of the highest quality, it is usually only applicable as a group average. When I am faced with an individual, a patient, with their own unique constellation of circumstances, even the most powerful science available struggles to answer basic questions: why do they feel like this? What made him do that? Why did this happen to her? At its most extreme, this explanatory gap can feel like a chasm. The twentieth-century philosopher–psychiatrist Karl Jaspers went so far as to describe it as an abyss.[2]

Into the Abyss is therefore not a mountaineering guide, although that *is* a good metaphor for my work. It suggests something that can be seen but is out of reach. It suggests dangers, darkness below. According to Jaspers, the abyss is an impenetrable country which separates 'us' from understanding the mind of the 'mad' or 'insane'. To me, the word 'abyss' implies a warning and a declaration of impotence. But it is also a challenge.

My first psychiatric hero was R.D. Laing, the radical Glaswegian thinker of the 1960s and 1970s. Initially Laing was an admirer of Jaspers, but later he became convinced he could connect even with the most disturbed people, those whose contact with reality is the least secure.[3] For Laing, the impediment to bridging this chasm was objectivity – the very stance that defines the scientific method. I used to fancy myself as a radical and might have followed in Laing's footsteps, but it wasn't really me. I suppose I am too fond of the firm footing provided by empiricism and cautious inference. This is what my training in one of the United Kingdom's most eminent psychiatric institutions gave me – although it hasn't stopped me at least trying to figure out what's going on in another person's mind.

Jaspers made a useful distinction between a 'meaningful' and 'causal' understanding of human behaviour. Meaningful understanding is about sympathising and empathising, telling stories, working back from the present to our formative experiences, as if they lie on a single, uninterrupted arc. But this powerful and occasionally beautiful way of seeing our lives may also be illusory: our lives are constantly buffeted about by the causal effects of DNA and disease and even chance. To put it another way, there are lots of things happening to us whether we believe in them or not.

Modern psychiatry is right to look to neuroscience for answers to some of the questions around human nature, and as a neuropsychiatrist, that has been my orientation. Yet some neuroscience – modern psychopharmacology, for example – has a lot to answer for. Neurotransmitters, biochemical messengers in the brain, are often described as the modern equivalent of the ancient humours. Just as the ancient Greeks held that blood and bile drove sanguine and melancholic temperaments, now we have dopamine and serotonin; the former, we are told, gives us motivation, and the latter is responsible for our moods. Then there is the adrenaline 'rush' and the endorphin 'high' and many more.

When it comes to dopamine, too little of it and you have Parkinson's disease; too much, and you have schizophrenia. So what about the patient described in chapter 1 who suffers from both? Understanding her condition is impossible without understanding the role of dopamine, but it is her shaky experience of the world, shaped and distorted through this chemical imbalance, that will expand rather than reduce our view of her.

One inescapable biological reality is the lump of fatty material sitting serenely in its protective casket on our necks. Solid and yet delicate, the brain is supremely vulnerable and the skull affords only modest protection. It is certainly no match for, say, a car speeding towards you. Having survived a traumatic brain injury you would hopefully, like the man in chapter 2, embark on a journey of recovery – as would your brain. It might seem hopelessly dualistic to separate the body and self in this way. We take our raw perceptions and intuitions as given; moment by moment, we have no awareness that there is a brain behind all this, doing the thinking. While philosophers have for centuries picked away at the illusion of unity, it is often only with damage to the brain that we start to notice the join, to see the 'bio' and the 'psycho' pulling apart. The patient's assumptions and expectations may not quite tally with the social and material world as their malfunctioning brain struggles to make sense of the disparity. Sometimes, it is only when we look at brain anatomy that we can make sense of a person's idiosyncratic reactions to injury. Maybe there is not such an abyss of understanding after all.

If the overall aim of this collection is to bridge the gulf of understanding between those with disorders and those without, a strong implicit theme rumbles on throughout: the tension between the perspective of an individual and that of the broader social world. For example, the presence of seismic social forces, such as racism and racial identity, can be heard loudly inside and outside the hospital and consulting room, as we see in chapter 4. In the face of prejudice, an individual might swing between extremes of mood until he finds a stabilising centre of gravity, a more natural rhythm and a familiar comforting tune in the therapeutic relationship. But does this relationship not perpetuate the same asymmetries of power? Another powerful social force is the imposition of expectations on women's bodies and the ethics of consumption, which surface in the clinic as 'eating disorders'. In chapter 5 we explore how these expectations, underpinned by the biological imperatives of hunger and reproduction, can become internalised across the life cycle, along with the body image inside our heads. But if society can talk us into it, there's a chance we can talk ourselves out of it.

The tension between the individual and wider society is especially evident when one tries to confront suicide. After all, it was the study of suicide in relation to culture and demography at the end of the nineteenth century that launched sociology as an academic discipline. If we go back to our newspapers, we will tend to find a faux consensus that suicide, being twice as common in men as in women, is due to a 'crisis in masculinity' and a culturally imposed ban on men talking about their feelings. Larger social factors, such as unemployment, alcohol and drug misuse, tend to be ignored, as does the single biggest risk factor: having a psychiatric disorder. Suicide fills the canon of our most revered literature. It litters Shakespeare's plays – think of *Hamlet, Macbeth, Romeo and Juliet,* and *Antony and Cleopatra.* Yet far from being a matter for introspection, the most effective suicide prevention tends to work at the population level: switching from coal gas to natural gas; putting up barriers in underground stations; even restricting the sale of paracetamol in chemist shops. Suicide takes us from the sublime to the banal, from the broad sweep of history to the minutiae of the individual's lonely struggle. We can never really know why a person takes their own life. Perhaps that's why, as in chapter 3, we are compelled to tell stories about it.

When meaningful and causal explanations meet, there is inevitably a tension, but if they come face to face in the same room, it can feel like an outright collision. It would be easy to claim that when this happens in the consulting room, the hapless psychiatrist is just an innocent bystander. That would be letting us off too easily as well as diminishing our contribution. Others have gone further to say that psychiatry is part of the problem, an agent of the state, a literal 'thought police'. The charge is excessive, but there is some circumstantial supportive evidence: we alone among medical practitioners have powers to detain and to coerce. We can force treatment on those who would refuse (chapters 1, 4 and 6); we can separate people from their families. In truth, the psychiatrist upholds society's norms and values, but he or she must not be a passive vector for these, let alone a salesperson. We are not required to be faceless and anonymous like the caricature psychoanalyst. Equally, we can't disguise our gender, race, class or the powers we have been given. And if we hide behind these attributes, we won't even see the space between us as persons, let alone bridge it. Writing of tension and collisions sounds rather negative, and not all the endings are happy ones, but these words speak to a potential energy which can be transformational.

The final chapter (chapter 7) picks up the threads of themes sounded earlier in the book through the stories of two people I met at a similar time. As it turns out, their quite different stories encapsulate much of the journey that mental health research and practice has travelled in the past century (and indeed from antiquity). As well as the humours, the ancient Greeks had some pretty odd ideas about the role of organs such as the womb, and how this might cause in women an affliction known as 'hysteria'. It was this condition that lured Sigmund Freud away from pursuing a stable and respectable career as a neurologist into the altogether more uncertain and, at times, sexually charged realm of mental disorder. A century later, we are still struggling with the same dilemmas and uncertainties that he was.

The last chapters in this book are about how brain and mind interact and, in a sense, vie for control. This can create intimate family dramas – as well as be provoked by them – which play out in the theatre of biomedicine. That brings us to the most potent and controversial symbol of treatment in psychiatry, and one which emblematises the clash between the physical and the metaphysical: electroconvulsive therapy (chapter 6), as well as its gentler modern cousin, transcranial magnetic stimulation (chapter 7).

All of the case histories herein are about how personal and shared beliefs can be powerfully destructive but can also help us to change for the better; one might even say they can be healing. I am aware that my account is partial and distorted by biases in recollection and exposition, as well as all the other influences that blindsided me at the time and, no doubt, still do. All of the chosen encounters were proverbial learning experiences and have helped me understand myself a little better (if no one else). Some readers will be aghast at my level of ignorance to start with. I am prepared to accept that; setting myself up for such judgements is not going to be comfortable, but it *is* necessary. On my side, or at least at my back, is the growing body of knowledge on mental health and illness. It is contained in the textbooks and academic journals rooted in both the biological and social sciences, a body of knowledge so vast that it can no longer be contained in a physical library.

My aim is to make use of some of this accumulated data (I prefer that to wisdom) without burdening the reader with too many citations. Much of it wags its finger at me admonishingly for being unread, while the rest is a reassuring presence – being there if needed. I mention this because I would also like to demystify psychiatry a little. It may be mysterious but it is not mystical; although, when it's just two people in a room, talking, it is sometimes amazing.

1

Dopamine

I first met Jennifer on an acute medical ward, lying in bed motionless. Literally motionless. She was lying on her back, slightly hunched forward, her head touching the pillow but not resting on it. She had a complicated, even contradictory, set of problems and had stopped taking her medication. She was losing weight and getting dehydrated. She had been admitted to hospital as an emergency.

Jennifer was in her mid-thirties. She was from a fairly ordinary middle-class family. Her parents separated during her childhood and she lived with her mother until her early teens, at which point her mother developed mental health problems and became increasingly paranoid and religiose, although she never saw a psychiatrist. From then, Jennifer started spending more time with her father. She was a good student and had won a place at art school. She took to photography and experimented with prolonged exposures of objects in motion (for example, trains passing, kids running and gliding birds), all of which produced unsettling blurry images. Midway through, when she was about twenty-one years old, Jennifer began to become paranoid, just as her mother was, convinced that people were stealing her ideas and possessions. She started to hear the voice of a famous film star who lived in her area. The voice said nasty, spiteful things and demanded that she cease painting or else… She felt compelled to obey such orders. He said he knew what she was thinking. There was also a female voice that she didn't recognise, and the two voices would speak to each other, commenting on what Jennifer was doing: "Look at her now, she's getting out of bed. Who does she think she is?" Bizarrely, the voices seemed to transform into the physical realm and invade her body, pulling at her sexual organs. These strange experiences are diagnostic symptoms of that most iconic mental disorder, schizophrenia.

She was seen by a psychiatrist at that time and, despite attempts to help her with medication and general support, she couldn't complete her art course. Without that major focus in her life, she became increasingly isolated, living alone in a bedsit on state benefits. She engaged only reluctantly with the local mental health team, tending not to trust them, but she did accept antipsychotic medication. It 'dampened down' the voices but didn't eradicate them.

In fact, she didn't really trust anyone. She believed that people entered her flat and went through her things, changed the furniture around and stole what few valuables she had. She took to going everywhere with a rucksack on her back stuffed with everything she owned, including letters, papers, CDs and sketches, so that they would be safe. Slung around her chest was a hefty, expensive but now battered camera. She behaved like a photojournalist without a subject, snapping frantically whenever she met someone or went somewhere new. The explanation was that she wanted to keep a record of her life so that she could, if need be, check up on what happened, who was there, where the objects were and so on, in order to use it as evidence. Evidence for what? Her defence? The prosecution? It wasn't clear.

In time, things settled down. Jennifer was looking after herself, venturing out to the shops to buy essential supplies, taking pictures from time to time and doing pastel self-portraits. She studiously avoided other people, but after many visits, a community psychiatric nurse began to establish a tenuous relationship with her. Over the next few years, they tried different medications to control her symptoms, but the clinical team were struck by the appearance of some very marked side effects. She complained that her movements were stiff and that she was dribbling excessively. She developed a tremor, especially in her right hand, which interfered with her drawing. It was as if, by blocking the crucial dopamine receptors in her brain, the antipsychotic medication had given her the symptoms of Parkinson's disease.

***

Antipsychotics were discovered in the early 1950s and hailed as the first drugs that could calm an individual without making them sleepy. One of the key areas of research was on the neurotransmitter dopamine, which attracted the attention of Arvid Carlsson, a Swedish pharmacologist working in the US National Institutes of Health. He showed that chemically induced depletion of dopamine led to loss of movement in experimental animals and he speculated that Parkinson's disease, the hallmark of which is a similar slowing of movement, may be caused by a lack of dopamine.[1]

It was well known that patients with Parkinson's disease showed degeneration of a small cluster of cells in the midbrain, called the substantia nigra because of its dark colour, which has a high concentration of the chemical neuromelanin, a precursor of dopamine. Those cells feed into the basal ganglia, which is crucially involved in movement control and contains high concentrations of dopamine. The basal ganglia are a small collection of neurones (ganglia) on either side, deep in the base (basal area) of the brain. Experimental and clinical studies in the early 1960s gave doctors the ability to replace the lost dopamine in Parkinson's patients, and the treatment showed dramatic benefits. It became the established treatment for what was previously an untreatable condition, and for his work Carlsson went on to share the Nobel Prize in Physiology or Medicine in 2000.

Over the same time period, a drug called chlorpromazine started to be used as a 'tranquilliser' for people with schizophrenia. For the first time, here was a treatment that was really effective at reducing psychotic symptoms, but doctors noticed that it produced side effects that were reminiscent of Parkinson's disease. And so we began to see the two diseases as mirror images of each other: schizophrenia was due to too much dopamine in key areas of the brain, whereas Parkinson's disease was due to too little. That theory, the original version of the dopamine hypothesis of schizophrenia, still accounts for many of the facts around schizophrenia. For example, most drugs which produce schizophrenia-like effects have been shown to act via an increase in dopamine transmission and, conversely, most drugs with antipsychotic effects do the opposite: they block or deplete the amount of dopamine in the brain.

We can think of neurotransmitters as being like the baton in a relay race. Nerves convey information in the form of electrical impulses. This is like the runner taking off down the track. Once they reach the end of their leg, they need to pass the baton to the hand of the next runner. The gap between the two runners is analogous to the synapse, a tiny cleft between two nerves. Once the new nerve is safely in receipt of the baton, the message is able to continue further. As in a relay race, this is a point where flow can be enhanced or disrupted. In Parkinson's disease there just aren't enough runners carrying the dopamine baton and not enough batons reach the destination. Dopamine-replacement therapy is like putting out extra batons at the changeover point, increasing the chances that some will get picked up. Other dopamine-enhancing therapies prevent the breakdown of dopamine at the receptors – a bit like allowing stray batons to 'stay live' even if dropped, and permitting runners to pick them up.

With schizophrenia, each runner is carrying too many batons, making the changeover chaotic. Many 'messages' are being passed on even without being officially part of the race; the person has perceptions of things that are not really there. Antipsychotic agents are thought to work by blocking the receptors, either by giving fake batons (which don't count) to the receiving runner or, according to another version of the theory, loosening the binding of dopamine onto the receptor – coating the hands of the receiving runner in grease so that they drop the baton.

If it is all about an excess or a lack of dopamine, we would expect that medications to treat Parkinson's disease run the risk of causing schizophrenia-like symptoms and that antipsychotic medications are liable to produce parkinson*ism*, the symptoms of Parkinson's disease. But over the years, the theory has started to creak under the weight of evidence that doesn't quite fit. In fact, it has proved quite hard to show that all patients with schizophrenia have an excess of dopamine, and not all patients respond to dopamine-blocking drugs.[2]

One early challenge to the theory was the rare case of a patient who had Parkinson's disease *and* schizophrenia. Surely, you can't have both too much dopamine and too little? Tim Crow, a prominent psychiatry researcher, published a series of four cases in 1976 in which the patients had all developed Parkinson's disease many years before developing psychosis.[3] None was being treated with dopamine replacement or enhancement at the time the psychosis emerged, so according to the theory, what was happening should have been impossible. Perhaps schizophrenia and Parkinson's disease were not two extremes on a single, neat spectrum, but something altogether more complex.

***

Jennifer had responded moderately well to antipsychotic medication but seemed to be developing unusually severe parkinsonism, her hands shaking constantly beyond her conscious control. Her clinical team were concerned and started, slowly and cautiously, to reduce her medication. Jennifer could not have been more pleased given that she never really liked taking her tablets and now felt horrible. The team thought that they were simply dealing with side effects and that they could reach a happy medium with the minimum effective dose of medication – just enough to control the symptoms of hallucinations and paranoia without slowing her down noticeably. What followed was a rather difficult couple of years. Predictably perhaps, reducing her medication meant a return to her conviction that she was being followed and persecuted, and as a result she shut herself away and even hid from her community psychiatric nurse (CPN) when she came round to visit. Not only that, the reduction in medication led to only minimal improvement to her movements. It became increasingly difficult for the team to maintain any kind of contact with Jennifer. Coming off all medication, her mental state was deteriorating and her physical state was worsening as well. Her movements were sloth-like, and she walked with a stooped posture like a woman twice her age.

Having been 'stuck' in this unfortunate condition for several months, her consultant psychiatrist sought my opinion and we agreed that her case was unusual and that it might be useful for her to get an expert neurological assessment. After much persuasion, she agreed. The neurologist examined Jennifer and admitted her to the general hospital for some tests. Eventually, after much prevarication, the consultant was forced to at least entertain the idea that she might actually be suffering from

Parkinson's disease as well as schizophrenia; after all, she had been off all medication for over a year by that point. If it was merely drug induced, it surely would have improved a lot more by that point.

The tests included a dopamine transporter scan. This involves injecting a tiny amount of a radioactive tracer into the patient's vein, which allows us to see the special transporter proteins that tidy up stray dopamine molecules when we do the scan. In a healthy brain, there is supposed to be a 'hot spot' showing a concentration of dopamine transporter in the basal ganglia. It should appear as normal for people who have only drug-induced symptoms of Parkinson's, whereas people with real Parkinson's disease have a weaker and cooler hot spot. Early in the disease, production of the transporter falls; after all, you don't need so many transporters if the amount of dopamine has dropped dramatically. Jennifer's scan showed a significant cooling of the hot spot. Furthermore, the scan was asymmetrical, with more loss on the left side of the brain (which controls the right side of the body), which tallied with her worst symptoms. An asymmetrical scan is typical of Parkinson's disease, especially early on, due to degeneration of the substantia nigra starting on one side first, and counts against any drug-induced or toxic effects since these would be expected to affect all regions equally.

The neurologist concluded that Jennifer must have a form of Parkinson's disease that was not simply drug induced, although it might have been drug *triggered*; that is, she may have been vulnerable to developing Parkinson's disease at some point in the future, but exposure to antipsychotic, dopamine-blocking drugs probably brought this point much closer. (This is just a hypothesis and there isn't as yet good evidence to show that this can actually happen.) Most people develop Parkinson's disease in their sixties and seventies, but in rare cases it can affect young adults. In these early-onset cases, there may be a family history of the condition and predisposing genes are often found. Neither of these circumstances applied to Jennifer.

Not surprisingly, Jennifer became increasingly despondent, then depressed, then suicidal. She was now hearing voices almost continuously – haranguing her, telling her what to do, including urging her to kill herself. Working with the neurologist, we offered Jennifer some medications which improve some of the symptoms of Parkinson's disease without acting through the dopamine system. Such drugs, known as anticholinergics, are mostly effective early in the disease. They helped with the dribbling and tremor; however, the psychotic symptoms could not be ignored. Jennifer was so distressed by the hallucinations that she accepted the offer of new antipsychotic medication. This time we used a drug called clozapine which often works for 'treatment-resistant schizophrenia' and is one of the few drugs not to cause parkinsonism or to worsen Parkinson's disease.[4] Thanks to clozapine, anticholinergics and regular support from the community psychiatric team, who encouraged Jennifer to attend a day centre from time to time, she enjoyed a period of relative stability.

A few years went by and Jennifer's physical symptoms, particularly the slowing of movement, worsened, as would be expected in someone suffering from Parkinson's disease. Her neurology consultant added some very-low-dose levodopa (also known as L-DOPA): standard treatment for Parkinson's disease, it is the chemical which is converted to dopamine in the brain. The neurologist was worried that this would exacerbate the hallucinations and other symptoms. She was right.

Jennifer believed, with some justification, that she was a human guinea pig. We were nudging up the clozapine here, reducing L-DOPA there, tweaking the other meds, doing our best – but not really sure we were going to improve the situation. Jennifer started avoiding us. She would occasionally turn up at the day centre with her rucksack and camera, looking dishevelled and gaunt, and would disappear before we could make any plans to address her needs. The CPN would visit her flat, but often she did not answer the door; when she did, she would only get out of bed with huge encouragement. Her movements were painfully slow as if she was swimming in treacle. She would answer questions, but her voice became progressively weaker until it was just a whisper. Over about two weeks of this, she was barely eating, which was hardly surprising since it took her ages just to reach for a piece of bread and put it to her lips. The food would sit there unchewed, clogging up her mouth.

Then the nurse's visits met with no response. Mail was piling up outside. We were worried that Jennifer was not getting any medication for her Parkinson's disease, which could leave her physically unable to care for herself, even setting aside whatever preoccupations were going round in her mind. Where was she? Was she sleeping rough? Attempts were made to contact relatives, but they couldn't help. The mental health team were worried. What if Jennifer was in her flat but unable to answer the doorbell? They decided we had reached the moment of last resort and needed to break her door down in accordance with a section of the Mental Health Act, since it was quite possible that her health had deteriorated to the extent that her life was in jeopardy.

The team found Jennifer huddled on the floor with soiled clothes, conscious and awake but not speaking. Her limbs were flexed but held rigidly in position. Her pulse was thready; her mouth was dry. They called the ambulance and she was admitted straight away to a medical ward. The medical staff checked her over physically, washed her and gave her clean clothes. She was put on a drip and given antibiotics for a chest infection. Requests for consultations from the neurology and neuropsychiatry teams were made. The working diagnosis was expressed in that uniquely medical way with the question mark at the front: '?Catatonia'.

***

'Catatonia' is a broad term that encompasses a group of strange motor behaviours mainly characterised by lack of movement (or speech) or the maintenance of an abnormal posture. Descriptions in old textbooks talk of moving the person's limbs and them feeling like a tailor's dummy ('waxy flexibility') – staying in whatever position they are left in. Often the person stares ahead eerily, blinking infrequently. Some people use the term to describe brief instances of such behaviour, while I prefer to use it in a much more restricted sense when it dominates the person's appearance and behaviour and is sustained over several minutes, hours or even days. Other forms of catatonia describe when a patient who is otherwise mute repeats exactly what is said to them ('echolalia'), or the movement equivalent when, despite being otherwise motionless, they seem to mimic the examiner's actions ('echopraxia'). Catatonia is not a diagnosis in its own right and may be seen in people with schizophrenia but also severe affective disorder, when their mood is extremely low (as in stupor) or extremely high (as in mania). It can also occur as a reaction to extreme stress or interpersonal conflict.

When a person recovers from catatonia, they sometimes tell you what it was like. One patient told me that he had thought he had a nuclear bomb inside his body and that if he so much as moved a muscle the whole world would be annihilated. Another patient felt she was in a union with God and was in a state of ecstasy. Other patients have little or no recollection of being catatonic. Indeed, it is very likely that many such cases are not really 'psychiatric' but are the result of an abnormal brain state which, while different from, say, a coma or partial coma (which causes an abnormal pattern of brain waves as measured by a standard electroencephalogram and therefore can be easily excluded), is nevertheless due to a subtle alteration in brain chemistry or possibly even a rare form of encephalitis.[5] One neurochemical cause goes under the rather sinister-sounding label 'neuroleptic malignant syndrome'. This is caused by an unpredictable and idiosyncratic reaction to neuroleptic drugs (the original name for antipsychotic medication). With the older antipsychotic drugs, it probably occurred in as many as 3 in 100 patients, but with the modern, somewhat gentler drugs it affects more like 1 in 10,000 patients. It is thought to be due to an extreme sensitivity to the dopamine-blocking action of the drug such that there is an almost complete shutdown in dopaminergic activity, which can be fatal. It can also happen when people with Parkinson's disease suddenly stop taking their medication.

***

It was on the medical ward that I saw Jennifer, face to face, for the first time. Yes, she *was* catatonic. And she seemed petrified. I pulled the curtains round her bed and sat on a chair next to her. I introduced myself in as benign and reassuring a way as I could. I sat and watched and waited. She was skin and bone, and rather clammy. Her face showed little expression and seemed to be coated in a thin film of grease. It was 'mask-like' as described in the textbooks.

"How are you?" I said.

Nothing. She stared upwards, hardly blinking.

"You seem very frightened," I said.

She closed her eyes slowly. A tiny pool of sweat had gathered in the u-shaped indent at the top of her sternum. I dabbed it with a tissue and gently placed my hand on her wrist.

"You're safe now. I think you got like this because you stopped all of your medication. Once you get back on it you will start to feel better. I promise."

Just then, her lips showed a flicker of movement. Was she trying to say something? I leaned in.

"Say again, Jennifer."

A murmur, slightly stronger this time.

"Sorry, I still can't quite hear you. Please try again," I urged, leaning closer.

Her eyes opened and she seemed to be summoning every effort to communicate.

"Once more – nearly there," I said as I bent down, my ear close to her lips.

"Let…go…of…my…arm."

It was barely a whisper. I drew back.

"So sorry, I didn't mean to…"

I was reminded that Jennifer was not an ordinary person who had succumbed to a serious illness and would be expected to passively and gratefully receive her treatment. She was someone who followed her own rules. She was a unique individual: suspicious, sparing in trust, preferring to be independent and rely on her own sources of information to determine the truth. She had suffered physically from an unlucky vulnerability to medication and a disorder most often afflicting the elderly. She had also suffered mentally from the illness which she may have inherited and which brought with it persecutory voices that followed her around, invading her body most intimately, invading her very being, her self, her private thoughts.

***

Should a male psychiatrist ever touch his patient? 'No' would be my answer most of the time but perhaps not always. The psychiatric consultation does occasionally give way to egregious violations of the doctor–patient relationship. The setting is private, contact prolonged, the emotional tone heightened and the power imbalance usually obvious. I don't believe in the total absence of personality in the consultation, as you might see in the ultra-formalism of psychoanalysis where the analyst is more or less invisible and certainly untouchable. I sometimes shake hands on first meeting, but only if the patient wants to. A paranoid person may feel attacked or cornered, and someone with obsessions or fears of contamination will recoil and worry that they may have suffered some detrimental contact and start ruminating on that before you've even started. But what of the person who is visibly upset and tearful, for example, recalling a bereavement or other loss? Surely it doesn't hurt to reach out a hand and connect, or give a brief hug on the way out? It may seem like the right thing to do. There is no injunction to be cold and distant; detached yes, aloof no. I often observe less experienced colleagues, when dealing with a patient who starts to cry, becoming animated, seeking the box of tissues, reaching out to comfort for fear of being seen as unempathic and then getting into a rather stereotyped duet where the patient, trying to compose themselves, says, 'Sorry, I shouldn't...' and the colleague offers the stock response: 'No, not at all'.

Like anybody else, it's not that I like seeing people weep or break down. It's just that I have learned to suppress a need – my need – to shut it down. I usually find myself leaning forwards, looking attentively at the person and trying my best to find something useful to say that isn't a cliché. Sometimes reaching out a hand at this point feels OK to me. But let's not kid ourselves: if that's all it took to lift a person out of their distress, they would likely have been reassured and comforted long ago – they wouldn't need to see a psychiatrist. When people are very seriously depressed, they don't cry much. They've passed that point.

The episode with Jennifer made me reflect on this and notice the subtle transformation that occurs when, as a neuropsychiatrist, I cross the road from the psychiatric hospital to the general hospital – alien territory. In the latter there is a lot of touching. The various rituals of pulse taking, listening to the heart, brow mopping and, in neurology, limb flexing and reflex tapping, all facilitate human contact. Funny, then, that other medics sometimes denigrate psychiatry as being all 'touchy-feely'.

It used to be that you could tell the senior hospital consultants apart by their dress code. They were invariably male, wearing white coats, smart suits and bow ties: proper doctors. The 'psychs', on the other hand, were all crumpled corduroy or loose dresses and sensible shoes. Then hospital infection control became the watchword and out went the white coats, to be replaced by shirtsleeves above the elbow, disposable aprons and plastic gloves. Psychiatrists were slow to fall in line and, for a brief spell, in our jackets and ties, or trouser suits, we were somewhat better dressed than our physician and surgeon counterparts. My comeuppance came when an officious ward matron narrowed her eyes, pointed and said, '*That* is a lethal weapon'. I looked down thinking I must have left my flies undone. She was referring to my tie.

***

Jennifer was in hospital for several months. It took a long time before she was able to even swallow food, so she had to be fed through a tube. Getting the right balance of medications was exceedingly difficult with her swinging between psychosis and excessive movements or, on the other hand, grinding to a parkinsonian halt. I observed other doctors, including my neurology colleagues, testing the tone in her muscles to gauge parkinsonian stiffness. She didn't recoil, but I could tell that she was not comfortable with physical contact.

I got to know her gradually. She wasn't easy to talk to. Many times she would just turn away. Sometimes I persisted, but I realised this was not a good approach. It was better to just sit there; eventually, she began to say a few words. She had a wry sense of humour ("You again! Run out of patients to see?"). Sometimes she would give me snippets of the gossip she over- heard from the general nurses while they attended to her 'personal care' – nurses who would forget that she was fully conscious and alert. Other times, however, she would despair, tears oozing from her unblinking eyes.

"Is it the voices again?" I would ask. "Yes," she would say, but then nothing more. Once she said, after a long silence, "Why are they torturing me?" At least I think that's what she said. It might have been, "Why are *you* torturing me?"

After the long process of physical recovery, Jennifer was transferred to an inpatient neuropsychiatry ward. Thanks to the combined efforts of the National Health Service at its best, with specialists in neurology, gastroenterology and general medicine, and with sustained input and care from nurses, doctors, physiotherapists and many others, she had come back

from the brink of death to a point where she was able to participate in more comprehensive rehabilitation. This included
regaining strength and becoming more mobile until she was
walking around almost normally with just the hint of a shuffle.
Fine tuning of medication enabled her to eat and talk with
ease. She was subject to 'on–off' phenomena, well recognised
in Parkinson's disease. This means that rather than symptoms
beginning to build up as the dose of the last medication wears
off, there is an abrupt transition from the individual feeling
their limbs to be loose and flexible, to completely seizing up.
Spreading out the medication into small but frequent doses,
every three hours, can alleviate this, although it puts a burden
on the patient and their carers to adhere to such a regime. That
might be a problem for Jennifer when she was discharged, but
she was nearly there. She was no longer the frail young waif,
lying in a hospital bed, depending on others to be bathed and
fed, inevitably infantilised, being visited upon by medical
professionals. Now she was able to inhabit fully the body of a
young woman, to express her hopes and aspirations, to seek
company and solitude as and when she pleased.

As for her psychotic symptoms, they were in abeyance
thanks to the clozapine. The voices, including that of the film
star she thought she knew, were still around and Jennifer
sensed his malign presence from time to time, but she felt
strong enough to defy him. She also described the phenomenon that, although her movements were much smoother, she
nevertheless experienced the sensation that they were not
always wholly under her control. She described this as if she
was a camera being manipulated by people in an outside

studio, zooming in here, panning to the left, tilting to the right... She thought 'he' was behind it but couldn't be sure. Psychiatrists call this 'passivity', a classic symptom of schizophrenia, and it means the person feels that their body (and mind) is the passive victim of outside influence, that they are not party to it, and they cannot resist.[6]

One thing that was important to Jennifer was artistic expression. Psychiatric rehabilitation units, when adequately funded, employ occupational therapists and sometimes art therapists. In the unit I worked on we were lucky enough to have a variety of highly skilled therapists who were full of initiative and always looking for ways to engage patients and work collaboratively with them. For someone whose ability to express herself was so often stymied, Jennifer eagerly made use of the facilities available, which included a well-stocked art room. The staff worked with all the patients on the unit as well as local organisations and volunteers to put on an exhibition. Jennifer was in her element. As well as producing some new works – portraits of other patients and self-portraits – she dug out some of her old pictures and photos, and framed them. I felt proud of her.

The exhibition took place one sunny summer's day in the occupational therapy department. Many people came – patients, friends, family, staff and members of the public. Lots of the items were for sale. One picture caught my eye. It was one of Jennifer's photographs using prolonged exposure. The scene, barely discernible, was a fairground at night. The technique produced a vibrantly coloured but shaky image of what might have been dodgem cars or a roller coaster, with lines of electric light smeared across it. Camera shake. Parkinson's.

How fitting. I asked how much it was. Eighty quid. A bit steep, I thought. Surely after all we've been through, the months of painstaking care, the time spent at the bedside, the shared satisfaction of gradual recovery, she'd give me a discount... She fixed me in her stare, unsentimental, inscrutable.

I handed over the money.

2

Strawberry Fields Forever

Patrick was a fitness fanatic and sports enthusiast. Recently married and a successful journalist, his life was shattered the instant he was thrown off his bicycle, hit from behind by a van travelling at 50 mph. It was thought that Patrick may have intended to turn right. Perhaps the van driver didn't see his signal or maybe took a chance and tried to overtake him. The result was that Patrick somersaulted backwards over the bonnet and 'bull's eyed' the windscreen. He was rushed to hospital and taken to the intensive care unit unconscious. A brain scan showed multiple cerebral contusions (bruises on the brain) and he had a broken arm. People kept saying that despite his injuries, he was lucky to have survived at all.

After about a week, he started to come round. He had no recollection of the actual accident. Although able to speak and move his limbs, he was weak down his left side and was confused – unable to remember what day it was, where he was or how he got there. After about a month, he began to participate in rehabilitation. Superficially he seemed to be getting back to normal very quickly, and in many ways he was the perfect patient: at thirty-two years old, he had been in good physical shape; fit, intelligent and by all accounts a really nice guy; not a thrill seeker, no alcohol or drugs, no previous psychiatric history. He worked hard and cooperated with the physiotherapists.

It wasn't all plain sailing. His memory let him down at times, and he would ask repeatedly where he was. He found it difficult to hang on to complicated instructions (do this, and when you've done that, do the other). He would lose track, get frustrated and could become morose. Months went by, and physically he was able to do almost everything he had done before: he could walk, jog and even ride a bike. But mentally things weren't quite right. He seemed unusually perplexed. He could tell you the time and date, where he was, the name of the hospital ward, who he was and the names of his therapists. But from time to time he would look at them quizzically and say things like, "Is this really happening? It doesn't feel real." They responded by trying to reassure him. After all, he was recovering from a serious accident. He could have been killed. That's bound to leave you shaken. Who in Patrick's situation would not ask themselves questions about reality, and even what life itself means?

In time, he was well enough to return home, coming to the rehab centre twice a week. His wife, Vicky, was very supportive. Everyone agreed they were a lovely couple. She worked in TV. She had a bubbly personality and was trying her best to be upbeat and positive, but she was beginning to feel the strain. Patrick had changed. He was glum, lacking in motivation and given to sudden losses of temper. His appetite and sleep were poor, and he had let himself go, washing irregularly and showing no interest in how he looked, nor in their new home. Vicky tried to give him space and they stopped sharing a bed. The couple were told by the hospital staff that all this was to be expected after a serious head injury. But there was something else going on, and Vicky was determined to get to the bottom of it.

One day she dug out some of their wedding photos and brought them along to the rehab centre. She wanted people to know that the person they were dealing with day to day was not the real Patrick – the pictures couldn't lie. In the photos Patrick was handsome, engaged, attractive and, judging by the expressions on the faces of those around him, witty and entertaining. This was the man she fell in love with. The staff gathered round and gushed – didn't they both look beautiful? And everything would be fine. They just had to be patient. It's a healing process; it takes time.

Not only did this fail to cheer up Patrick, it seemed to drive him into an even greater despair. That evening he confronted Vicky. Why did she bring those stupid photos to the rehab centre? What was she trying to prove? And then the bombshell: "You're not even my wife. You're not the real Victoria." It all came spilling out. Ever since the accident he'd had the feeling that something wasn't right. Things around him seemed strange, ineffably different. He wasn't the same either. It wasn't just that he bore the scars of the injury, it was something much more profound. He wasn't even convinced he was alive. Maybe he had died in the accident; after all, how many people survive being knocked off their bikes by a van going 50 mph? It made just as much sense that this was a kind of afterlife or purgatory. The people he used to know had been replaced by imposters using their bodies as 'shells'. Of course he couldn't sleep with this woman; that would be committing adultery. He loved the *real* Vicky – she must be somewhere – and he wasn't going to betray her.

Vicky was stunned. How ironic that she had brought the wedding photos to show people 'the real Patrick'. Naturally, there is more to a person than can be conveyed by a snapshot, a glossy image caught in time. But it turned out that for different reasons, they had both been worrying about what had happened to 'the real Patrick'. In a very deep sense, Patrick *had* changed. It's not just that following the accident he was injured; in *his* mind he was fundamentally different and, specifically, negated. He had become unreal and with him the world too was unreal.

The next few weeks were awful. Vicky would try to reason with Patrick, but it got nowhere and only ended in rows. From Patrick's point of view, any new evidence confirmed that there had been an alteration of everything he thought he knew and valued. He felt deeply alone and realised that what he was going through was outside the realm of normal experience. He couldn't carry on like this. One night he barricaded himself in the spare room. When Vicky eventually broke the door down she found Patrick slumped in a chair. He had sprayed fly killer into a cup and tried to drink it. She dialled 999.

Patrick was admitted to the local psychiatric hospital. He was diagnosed with severe depression. He had all the signs, not least a profoundly low mood amounting to despondency, an attempted suicide, a lack of motivation as well as poor appetite and sleep. A full house. The psychiatrists called it 'psychotic depression', meaning that there was also evidence of delusions and hallucinations. He had lost contact with reality.

***

Hallucinations are defined simply as 'perceptions without an object', perceptions that cannot be put down to dreaming or transitions into and out of sleep, and are not believed to be under the person's control. Delusions can also be defined simply as false beliefs, but as soon as you start to think about it – and psychiatrists and philosophers have been for hundreds of years – you find that such a definition is really unsatisfactory.[1] First, what if your belief turns out to be true? You thought your partner was having an affair and you admit you had absolutely no evidence to support this, so it was a delusion. It later turned out that they *were* having an affair, so it wasn't a delusion. The solution to this is to say that a delusion is an unfounded belief. So far, so good. But what if I believe that I am going to captain England in the World Cup? Maybe it's a daydream, a fantasy, wishful thinking perhaps, but a delusion? That seems to go too far. If you ask me whether I seriously believe this, I will concede it's not going to happen

– but it's not logically impossible.[2] So what about someone who says they believe in a supernatural being that created the universe? Are they deluded, since there is no concrete evidence for this idea? Labelling this sort of belief as a delusion would not be a good move. As evolutionary biologist Richard Dawkins knows, it does make for an arresting polemic, but it also pathologises an awful lot of otherwise healthy people.

No, the definition of delusions has to have the proviso that the belief, while firmly held, is not widely shared or attributable to common cultural values. Even then, what about beliefs that are not shared and which, by their nature, are neither provable nor refutable? If someone said that the world was doomed, what kind of evidence could there be to back this up? Knowing some facts about our planet, you might conclude that it was true or, based on equally respectable knowledge, that it was false, or that you just couldn't say. Some beliefs are value judgements and are therefore subjective.

If someone says they are a bad person, could this be a delusion? In psychiatry, such a belief might be seen as a symptom of depression where negative self-evaluation is the hallmark, and if it was extreme you might say it was a delusion. Here you would call on other factors which, strictly speaking, have nothing to do with epistemology – the truth of the statement itself – but the secondary effects which accrue *around* the belief. If the belief that you were a bad person was overwhelming, unshakeable, preoccupying, distressing, leading you to want to end your life, then surely it's 'abnormal' or 'pathological'.

So where does that leave us with our definition? A delusion is a fixed, unfounded belief that is not shared by a person's cultural milieu, and which affects the individual (and perhaps others) adversely. It may or may not be logically impossible. It may or may not be a matter of values rather than facts. That's about as good a definition as you can get.

Sometimes a particular delusion acquires a special status, usually because it keeps cropping up. Give the delusion a memorable name and its posterity is assured. Working in Paris, the eminent psychiatrist of his day, Joseph Capgras, and his assistant published in 1923 a detailed case study of a woman who had elaborate beliefs that certain people around her were not who they claimed to be, in particular her husband. They called it *l'illusion des sosies*, referring to a Greek myth in which the god Hermes takes on the appearance of the lowly Sosias so that Zeus, king of the gods, can seduce her. This illusion of doubles soon became better known as the Capgras delusion or syndrome.

Several reports followed, each more dramatic than the last. Perhaps the most shocking was a case where the supposed double was decapitated in an attempt to reveal their non-human nature. Themes also emerged from several of these stories, such as the close relationship between the deluded person and the presumed imposter, but also the variety of things supposedly replaced by a fake or copy, from pets to spectacles. Another clinical factor emerged that many, though not all, cases had in common: the sufferer had some kind of brain injury or degenerative disease. Patrick certainly fitted the profile.

As if having one obscure French delusion is not enough, the delusion that one is dead also has a name. It is *le délire des negations*, usually translated as 'nihilistic delusions' or called Cotard's syndrome after Jules Cotard, another Parisian physician. He was more of a neurologist than a psychiatrist and described the first cases of this kind in the 1880s. The belief that one is dead or in a kind of living death is the core feature of the delusion, but there are others, such as beliefs about the body being empty or decaying and the world around them being parched and barren. The urge to end this state was also noted by Cotard from the outset, and often the individual feels that they need to be not just killed but annihilated, even immolated. The anguish that this state engenders must be truly terrifying, and Patrick seemed to be in its grip.

***

At this point, Patrick believed he had died and was in some intermediate state between life and death, a parallel world where real things had been replaced by imitations. There are some cultural resonances here; think of zombies and the undead, doppelgängers, *The Stepford Wives*, *The Truman Show* or *Synecdoche, New York*. But these aren't shared beliefs in the way that religious beliefs are. No one in Patrick's cultural milieu shared his beliefs, least of all his own wife. Saying you have died is a blatant paradox, and acting on such a thought with the intention to kill yourself is the enactment of such a transparent logical contradiction that merely considering it starts to undermine your sanity.

Patrick received excellent care from his local mental health unit. Hours were spent trying to understand his concerns and fears. Along with psychological therapy, he was offered treatments such as powerful antidepressant and antipsychotic medication. His mood did improve and the suicidal thoughts diminished. The staff gave him practical help to get back into his routines of washing, dressing, eating and even working. He and Vicky attended counselling and tried to find new ways to get along. They were helped to understand how brain injury can have an effect on all aspects of a person's life and well-being. After a long admission and subsequent outpatient care, one year on, the situation was stable but also stuck. Patrick had tried to do some work from home, writing, but found it hard to concentrate. Vicky was having to work long hours to pay the mortgage. Seeing each other less seemed to work for them. They avoided discussing the nature of reality and all the rest, since the conversation just went round in circles. Vicky couldn't empathise with whatever Patrick would say and this, in turn, just made him feel more isolated.

Patrick was referred to our neuropsychiatry service. I met him and Vicky and explained that I wasn't at all sure we would be able to offer much, but that we would do some investigations and try to take a fresh look at the problem. I was impressed by the couple's obvious affection for each other despite the barriers that Patrick's illness had put between them. I had

several conversations with Patrick after that and felt he was
someone with whom we could work. Yes, he had a slew of
bizarre, entrenched ideas, but he also seemed to be able to step
back a little and question them. I found him to be earnest and
dogged but willing to learn. How much this was his basic
personality and how much had been distorted by the brain
injury was hard to determine. He was the son of a schoolmas-
ter and prided himself on being methodical and 'doing his
homework'. He was a mine of information that seemed to
survive the other areas of memory loss. Dates and scores of
important sporting contests were still there, which was not
surprising for a sports reporter. Plus, he could explain in painstaking detail the strengths and weaknesses of, for example,
Shimano bicycle gears versus Campagnolos – to anyone toler-
ant enough to listen.

One question was how much brain damage Patrick had
suffered. We carried out a magnetic resonance imaging (MRI)
scan which, at this point, would show us the permanent effects
of the accident. (MRI produces a very detailed picture of the
structure of the brain including the white and the grey matter,
with resolution down to 1 or 2 mm.) It showed that there were
bad signs in both the white and the grey matter of his brain.
The white matter inside the brain is a bundle of connecting
fibres, each wrapped in an insulating layer of fat (myelin)
which speeds up transmission of electrical impulses. The grey
matter covers the outside of the brain like a thick, ruffled blanket. It comprises mostly cell bodies, the engine room of the
cell, and has a rich blood supply to bring in fuel and take away
waste products. It looks a kind of pinkish-grey in real life. Each

brain cell has connections going in and out, so under a microscope it looks a bit like an octopus.

There were fairly extensive lesions (i.e. scars) in the white matter, in the frontal lobes behind the forehead and the temporal lobes above the ears. Clearly the scan showed that some of the connections had been damaged. This could affect reasoning and perception. There was also evidence of old bruising – MRI can 'see' blood products because it picks up the iron content – in the grey matter, again in the frontal and temporal lobes, more so on the right. (This would explain why, at the very beginning, Patrick was weak down his left side.)

The MRI also showed that the sulci, the inner folds of the grey matter, were generally wider than would be expected for someone of Patrick's age, showing disruption to the brain and the death of nerve cells, which probably occurred on impact when Patrick came off his bike. The brain shrinks as we get older and, as it does, the sulci become wider and the gyri or outer folds become thinner (atrophy), so the overall folded appearance becomes more obvious. Patrick's brain looked like that of a man twice his age. The MRI also revealed that the inner part of the temporal lobe, including the hippocampus, a curl of grey matter tucked under each side, was smaller on both sides, meaning he would be expected to have an impaired memory.

The ward neuropsychologist also assessed Patrick. She gave him a battery of tests covering language, perceptions, memory and reasoning, designed to show problems or deficits in any of these functions. Neuropsychologists sometimes use these tests to infer where, in the brain, damage might have occurred to produce a particular pattern of deficits. In Patrick's case, the testing took several hours and had to be spread out over several days to get the best out of him and avoid fatigue. Interpreting the tests requires skill and training, and not just a little art. How the patient goes about doing the tests – solving the puzzle, remembering the list and so on – can be as revealing as the test scores themselves.

The tests showed that Patrick's overall IQ was pretty much back to the level you would expect for someone with his education and occupation. It was a remarkable story of recovery, given how serious his accident was. His basic visual perception was intact: he could copy shapes, name objects and distinguish between similar patterns. But there were some areas where he performed less well than he should have. His memory was OK, but when pushed he made mistakes. He was given a series of pictures (i.e. scenes) to look at one by one and then shown very similar scenes in pairs (one of which had been shown to him before). He was asked which one of them he recognised. If you guessed blindly, you would get 50% correct. Most healthy people get over 90% correct. Patrick performed much better than chance but below the healthy range.

There was one test with which he struggled: the Wisconsin Card Sorting Test. The test comprises a pack of cards, each of which has three dimensions: shape (square, circle, cross or star); number (up to four); and colour (red, green, blue or yellow). You start with four cards laid out side by side, for example, a red circle, two green stars, three yellow squares and four blue crosses. Your job is to say where the next card belongs in the sequence. Let's say you are shown a card with a yellow cross. You have a guess and place it next to the yellow squares (you're going with colour). But no – it's wrong. So you guess that it's about the shape. You place it on the one with the blue crosses. This time it's correct. The next run of cards are easy to sort; you just concentrate on shape. But suddenly the rules change. After some trial and error, you realise that the key sorting dimension is now number. So now you can ignore shape and colour and stick to number of items. And so it goes on. Where some people go wrong is that they take a long time to infer the 'sorting rule' and then they may forget what it is. But another problem occurs when, having got on to the correct rule, you stick to it even when you are being told your answers are wrong. You keep going for red when you should have switched to triangles. This is a more interesting kind of mistake. Psychologists call it perseveration and it is evidence of a wider problem in 'set-shifting'. This is traditionally attributed to damage to the frontal lobes.[3] The failure to shift set or think flexibly is a considerable handicap in the real world, where no one tells you the rules and, just when you think you've figured them out, they go and change them. Patrick struggled with this test and, not only that, he hated it. It wasn't fair!

Another domain of thinking where Patrick's abilities were tested was face processing. In fact, he recognised famous faces and was able to match photographs of faces of the same person taken at different angles. He did make some mistakes and spent ages going back and forth before deciding on the correct answer, whereas most people fly through it. By looking at how he answered, and not just whether he got it right, we could infer that there might be damage to the right hemisphere of the brain. Another test was of facial expressions. Facial expressions of emotions can be grouped together under a handful of major categories: happy, sad, angry, disgusted, surprised and fearful are considered the most basic. Patrick did fine on this test, except for expressions of fear. He consistently got it wrong and just couldn't seem to see the expression for what it was. This pointed to damage to the amygdala, a small structure next to the hippocampus, which is a critical hub in processing emotions.

The ward psychologist also gave Patrick some questionnaires with items about day-to-day behaviour, common difficulties and reactions, things like losing your temper easily, getting frustrated and being absent-minded. Patrick certainly ticked a number of the boxes where he had problems. What was particularly revealing was when Vicky filled out the same questionnaire giving her perspective on Patrick. There was a discrepancy over virtually all the answers. Patrick might say that he was 'occasionally' more irritable than he used to be, whereas Vicky said that it happened 'very often'. On other questions he failed to register that there was anything wrong while Vicky clearly noted a change for the worse. Patrick's consistent lack of insight into his own difficulties in thinking and social behaviour, such as failing to appreciate other people's feelings and acting impulsively, was exposed, as was the gulf in understanding between him and Vicky which was causing such strain in their relationship. This lack of insight is often attributed to deficits in frontal lobe or executive functioning (although I wouldn't necessarily advise couples with intact frontal lobes to carry out this exercise).

***

With most of the investigations out of the way, Patrick settled down and adjusted to the new ward. He began talking more openly about his worries and concerns. He still felt low but not without hope. I started to probe the topics that had been a 'no-go area' for Vicky. I was keen to try to see the world from Patrick's perspective. How could a person with his background and experience come to hold beliefs that were logically absurd?

I started with general questions about his overall mood and experiences. He described the pervasive sense of being changed, less vibrant, less in touch, and of the world itself being changed: it was flat, monotonous, like watching a movie or being in a fog. These descriptions were instantly recognisable as *depersonalisation* (where the person seems unreal) and *derealisation* (where the world seems unreal). Many healthy people describe similar feelings, especially when extremely fatigued or stressed (after childbirth, for example). This does not usually amount to a delusion because people preface their descriptions with 'as if': it's *as if* I am an automaton going through the motions; it's *as if* I am in a movie; it's *as if* I am behind a pane of glass. Depersonalisation and derealisation (the two tend to go together) have also been described following life-threatening danger. American psychiatrist Russell Noyes and psychologist Roy Kletti collected a number of first-person accounts of those who had survived near-death experiences, such as losing one's footing while mountaineering, and noted that people sometimes entered a rather unnerving state of calm. Often their senses are heightened, but they feel like a detached observer of their own drama. Perhaps it is an adaptive response, a safety mechanism,[4] like a valve opening which prevents the mind being overwhelmed by a surge of anxiety. But in those cases it's transient.

In psychiatry, depersonalisation and derealisation often accompany other more familiar symptoms of anxiety or depression, but they can still occur on their own as a primary disorder. It can be hard to recognise. People look fine from the outside and often don't want to talk about their situation for fear of being labelled. But they are really suffering inside. One sufferer describes it this way:

> If I quieten my mind, I can *almost* [emphasis added] taste the colour and richness of life as I knew it before... This is, I think, the very act of 'living', which I bear witness to in others, all day, every day. I still understand it academically, but I can barely remember what it feels like. These days I'm in a constant state of grief; I feel as if I'm grieving for my own death, even if I seem to be around to witness it.[5]

Some people seem to enjoy a state of mind which is a bit like this – detached, spacey – and they get it from commonly used drugs such as cannabis. Psychedelic drugs also do this as well as produce more dramatic distortions in perception. When John Lennon wrote that 'nothing is real' in 'Strawberry Fields' at the height of flower power in 1967, perhaps this was inspired by such drugs (or maybe just by enchanting childhood memories). Either way, it is not difficult to imagine that what may be a pleasant diversion for a few hours can become a deeply unpleasant cul-de-sac if it becomes enduring and uncontrollable – 'Strawberry Fields *forever*' – and this prolongation does happen, whether people have experimented with drugs or for no obvious reason at all. Depersonalisation and derealisation might appear as a safety mechanism, but in an unlucky minority, the valve 'blows' – maybe the surge of anxiety was too strong, or there was some physical change to the brain following an injury, and the state becomes fixed.

A lot of what Patrick articulated, both now and shortly after his head injury, seemed to be depersonalisation and derealisation minus the 'as if'. I asked him when he first gained the impression that the world was changed, false or unreal in some way. He vividly recalled coming back from the hospital for the first time after the accident. He was definitely not feeling great: he had a headache, his thinking was sluggish and he was full of trepidation. Sitting in the back of the taxi, he began to recognise the streets and landmarks of his hometown. But he pulled up short. That row of houses, where did they come from? They weren't here before. What was going on? It looked like his hometown but couldn't be; it was a fake, a trick, a forgery, and not a very good one.

I was taken aback. Haven't we all had the same experience? Not noticing a new block of flats in a place we haven't visited for a while? We register surprise but then accept that change happens; once contractors get going, modern buildings can go up pretty quickly. But while it seems obvious that things can look different in all sorts of ways and yet remain essentially the same, how this happens in the brain is not at all simple. In fact, scientists in artificial intelligence have been struggling with this problem for decades. Clearly memory cannot consist of a static record archive against which new perceptions are matched so that we can say, yes, I recognise that – it's my house, my street; no that's new, never seen that before. If it did, memory would keep failing as soon as the lighting was different or we were approaching the object from a different angle; or in the context of people, they had aged, changed their hairstyle, grown a beard and so forth. You would need an infinite number of versions for each memory record, and that would be so inefficient as to be impractical.

Of course, we do sometimes fail to recognise people if they change their look, at least initially and especially if we see them out of their usual context. Similarly, we do sometimes mistake a stranger for someone we know. That's because an efficient memory system must 'cheat' to some extent by building up expectations based on prior experience. An efficient memory system stores an abstract blueprint of the object that takes into account the ways it might change in time and context. Crucially, an efficient memory system must also be able to tolerate a margin of error: perhaps it's not quite what you were expecting, but it's close enough. Only recently have computers become able to recognise faces and voices, despite huge investment, and that's because software engineers have learned to copy the way our minds work.

Patrick had dozens of examples of uncanny memories, places and people that were almost right, but different.

"Why do you think the Vicky who visits most days is not the real Vicky?" I asked tentatively.

His eyes widened. "My Vicky, the old Vicky, she was very particular about her appearance. She had beautiful skin and great taste in clothes and make-up. She loved designer brands." He looked hesitant and started to blush, but continued. "She loved expensive underwear, you know, silk with lace. *Victoria's Secret*, that was our private joke… But this one…sure, she almost looks the part, but it's all Marks & Spencer's, baggy nylon, the elastic gone, washed-out colours."

He was deadly serious. I gently took this up with Vicky a few days later in a one-to-one session.

"Jeez! Doesn't he realise I have been working all hours to keep the house, to keep the show on the road while he's been in and out of hospital or up in his room staring into space? I can't *afford* to buy sexy underwear anymore, much as I'd love to."

***

This is the balancing act of our memory system: if my margin of error is too lax, then everything looks familiar even if I've never seen it before, and I will have constant *déjà vu*. If I am too strict, everything looks new, nothing looks familiar, I don't remember any of it, and I will be lost. What we have with Patrick is not quite that. Things *do* look familiar, but only up to a point. It *looks* like Vicky, but something is missing.

Recognition produces an emotional charge. In fact, we experience a physical response at the moment of recognition, especially when the thing or person is salient or emotionally resonant (like a loved one), and this can be detected in a laboratory as a skin conductance response (SCR). It is simply a tiny burst of sweat that increases the electrical conductivity of the skin, which is the basis of a lie detector test. When doing research in London, the Colombian psychiatrist Mauricio Sierra showed that people with depersonalisation disorder failed to show the usual SCR to emotional pictures compared with neutral ones.[6] He argued that this might lead them to develop the sense that things aren't quite real and that their emotions are numb, symptoms which go in tandem. But those suffering from depersonalisation disorder, who have such feelings most or all of the time, nevertheless do not think the world is actually different. They know that they and the world are real, despite how they feel. And they also don't show any obvious brain changes, damage or disease on their brain scans.

British neuropsychologists Hadyn Ellis and Andy Young proposed that what is happening in Capgras syndrome is not a simple problem in recognising people, but that the sufferer fails to get the reassuring pulse of recognition each time they encounter one of their nearest and dearest. The seeds of this are present in Capgras' original description:

> The feeling of strangeness is associated with recognition which conflicts with it. The patient, whilst picking up on a very narrow resemblance between two images, ceases to identify them because of the different emotions they elicit. Quite naturally she attributes to these similar beings, or rather to this unique, unknown personality, the name of doubles. With her, the delusion of doubles is not therefore really a sensory delusion, but rather the conclusion of an emotional judgement.[7]

But there's a problem here too. While that should lead to a sense of depersonalisation or derealisation (e.g. 'that's odd, it looks like my wife but something doesn't feel right'), why jump to the far-from-obvious conclusion that they have been replaced by a double or an alien? There must also be a reasoning failure. The initial error is skewed by the emotions and fears of the moment – a paranoid disposition – and then becomes entrenched by a lack of common sense.

Because of the brain injuries affecting his temporal and frontal lobes, Patrick had to work hard to match faces, so he may have been less accurate in his ability to recognise people and things under all circumstances. These perception regions were perhaps disconnected from emotion-generating areas, like the amygdala, because of white matter damage, so even when he recognised the look of his wife, he wasn't aided by a reassuring sense of familiarity. His memory was also not working perfectly due to damage to the hippocampus. Maybe he didn't automatically update memories to take account of natural changes to places (housing developments) and people (getting older and modifying their choice of clothes); instead, they were, in his mind, frozen at the time of his accident. He was able to learn and take in new information, but it took more effort than it should have and didn't happen naturally. He then lacked the facility to come up with reasonable explanations and test them out rationally, because of his frontal lobe damage. Once he latched on to an answer, *any* answer, he couldn't argue himself out of it, he couldn't shift set and he didn't see it as his problem because he lacked insight into his condition.

That still leaves the nihilistic delusions of Cotard, the feeling that one is already dead, unexplained – or does it? Andy Young and Kate Leafhead had noticed the coincidence of Capgras and Cotard delusions and came up with a nice explanation, which they generously credited to Cotard from his initial account.[8] The patient starts with various vulnerabilities: they may have suffered some brain injury, disease or chronic mental illness such that they struggle to process information and to reason flexibly and coherently. Then there is the critical defect in physiological feedback leading to an abnormal sense of unfamiliarity. The person with Cotard's syndrome is also severely depressed with a tendency to be self-critical, to blame themselves for everything; hence, the feeling that they are changed and lacking in vitality leads to the conclusion, obvious for them, that they must be dead, that the world is dead. It's an idea so overpowering that they find it hard to reason away. If, however, they are not in this negative self-blaming emotional state, but are of a rather more querulous disposition – it's someone else's fault; I'm the victim here – the same feelings lead to a different conclusion. It is the world that has changed and other people are not who they profess to be: Capgras syndrome. It's now not so difficult to see that the same person could oscillate between the two attribution states and, at different times, express both beliefs. That's where Patrick found himself.

***

With the help of the clinical team, the academic work of contemporary cognitive neuropsychiatry and a touch of creative speculation, Patrick and Vicky now had an explanatory model, which could make sense of the inexplicable. It was a good start, at least. The model allowed us to talk to each other about Patrick's experiences in a way that rendered them tractable, so that we could start unpicking the elements one by one. While this was going on we continued treating his depression with the usual methods and, as we predicted, the 'as if' seeped back in. That left the problems of thinking and reasoning, not least his propensity, when frustrated, to seek explanations in terms of shadowy outside forces. He stopped blaming himself but found it hard to take a middle road.

What if things just happen? They are no one's fault, there's no grand design, no plot. This is where the cognitive behavioural therapy (CBT) approach came in. CBT is all about pulling apart the thinking processes that lead to emotional reactions which, in turn, block cool rationalisation, leading to more frustration and so forth in a vicious cycle. Gradually, Patrick was taught to step back and examine his assumptions, to look out for conclusions driven by emotions and to force himself to go through problems logically and, if necessary, perform mini-experiments to gather data. For example, is there any other explanation for Vicky's uncharacteristic change in underwear choice? Was it correct to define her by this in the first place? What about economic factors?

Every time he experienced some doubt, a weird occurrence, something not quite right, some inauthenticity, he learned to write it down and force himself to generate alternative explanations, including that the world was unreal or fake. The therapist would then sit down with him and go through them methodically, systematically and without emotion until they could both agree on the most plausible one. Vicky started to take on the role of co-therapist. It was really working. He liked it. It suited his thinking style, his comfort in facts and consistency. He didn't need to be flexible, he needed to take one step at a time according to pre-agreed rules.

One session I had with Patrick was really memorable. We would often start off in the safest territory for a sports journalist: talking about football. The UEFA Football Championship had recently finished.

"So…" he began, "if the world is real and as it should be, how come Greece, a footballing minnow, won the European Championship? That just couldn't happen. They *apparently* beat Portugal, with Luis Figo, Cristiano Ronaldo, Nuno

Gomes…in Lisbon. They knocked out Holland! It doesn't make sense!"

I was taken aback. Again.

"Well, they had to beat teams to get to the final," I offered lamely.

"Yeah, Czech Republic," he sneered.

But the best teams don't always win. Even Manchester United didn't win the league that year, despite winning three out of the previous five seasons and, as it turned out, three out of the next five. Fortunately, Patrick by this stage was seeking a way of finding a different explanation and looked to me for guidance. We started thinking about sport and what made it so compelling. The victory for the underdog, the goal in injury time. This was just the sort of example that we could work on. A team's 'form' was all about setting up expectations. And when the expectations are dashed, you search for an alternative explanation. But sometimes there is no explanation, or at least not one with a narrative behind it with reasons and causes. Perhaps the most *common* reason for why something happens is the most difficult to accept. It's just chance, bad luck, or good luck, depending…

He wasn't entirely convinced. Fortunately, I found some evidence to back up my admittedly weak position. Some American theoretical physicists had recently published an article on, amazingly, the predictability of major sports.[9] Presumably, they were bored with uncovering the secrets of the universe. What they did was take the national league tables for American football, basketball, hockey, Major League Baseball and, finally, the English Football Association

(FA). Analysing masses of data from before 1900 to the present day, they looked at all the matches played and calculated the probability of the favourite (the team which at that point was higher in the league) winning the match. With some very complicated mathematics they were able to show that these sports could be ranked in order of their unpredictability (or competitiveness as they preferred to call it). American football was the least 'competitive' as the favourites usually won. English football was almost, although not quite, at chance level; that is, in any given FA league match, either team could win, even though overall the favourites just about come through on top.

It had been scientifically proven. Football is the best sport of all. It's the most competitive and unpredictable, and therefore the most exciting. It's not just down to chance; otherwise, there would be no point investing your devotion into one team or another. On the other hand, if your team always won, that too would be pointless and boring. No, the ideal sport is predictable enough so as not to be fickle, yet unpredictable enough to always have you on the edge of your seat, never knowing quite how it's going to end. That's what we love about sport. And that's what we should learn to love about life.

***

Patrick and Vicky went back home to the Midlands. Getting over a serious traumatic brain injury is slow and might never be complete, but they felt they could cope better now. Things were gradually improving. I lost touch with them but often thought about Patrick and how he would deal with the inevitable setbacks and surprises which life would throw at him, especially in May 2016. That month, the news came through of one of the most extraordinary, seismic and incredible shocks in the history of sport: Leicester City Football Club, having been in danger of relegation the previous season, and at odds of 5,000 to 1, were champions of the Premier League.

3

Losing My Religion

Depression is surprisingly common. Nowadays there is no shame in admitting you are among the one in six that have suffered from depression or are on antidepressants. Around 7.3 million people in the UK were prescribed antidepressants in 2017–18, over half of whom also received a prescription for such drugs in both of the previous two years.

Thomas led a quiet, undramatic life; he was privately a devout Christian. Married with two children whom he adored and a loving wife, he worked as a lorry driver. The road provided a certain peace; the solitude, the monotony, were plusses as far as Thomas was concerned. He had suffered a rather bad depressive episode three years back. There was no real reason, no obvious precipitant; he had what psychiatrists used to call 'endogenous' depression (literally 'produced within'). Thankfully, he had responded to antidepressants and returned to work. What he failed to do was inform his employer (and the Driver and Vehicle Licensing Agency) that he had been advised to continue with the medication. This was a serious omission. He was safe to drive – he was not erratic, suicidal or rendered drowsy by the medication – but if something happened and they found out, he could be in big trouble. Not only that, but he was lying and, in his world, that was a sin.

After a couple of years, the 'lie' started to bother him more and more. He was doing so well but he felt that, by lying, he had ruined it. He began to think that this always happened, that he never dealt with things properly, that he always took shortcuts. Thomas became tortured by these thoughts going round and round in his head and the conviction that he was a sinner in the eyes of God. People tried to reassure him, but it didn't help; in fact, that seemed to make it worse. He could see no escape from the thoughts or from his situation, and his mind turned to suicide. Why not? He was damned anyway.

I suggested to Thomas that he come into hospital, but he refused, saying there was no point, and that nothing would work. I took issue with that. He was the sort of patient who was likely to do well, to recover, given the right help.

***

What was it that was going on inside Thomas's head? It could be said that he was 'thinking too much' and was always assuming the worst. Not only that, we might question his interpretation of events. That is not to say that he was dissembling but that he was selective in his recall and somewhat one-sided; biased, in the terminology of cognitive psychology.

Cognitive theories of depression differ from broader psychological accounts in that they are less concerned with what you're thinking than how you're thinking. Most people's common-sense views of depression come from experiences of loss. Sigmund Freud put this together in an article entitled 'Mourning and Melancholia' published in 1917,[1] in which the experience of bereavement was compared with that of depression and the overlap pointed out. People with depression, it is assumed, must have suffered more than their share of losses – including the loss of work, health or more symbolic and abstract losses such as those of status and esteem. Social psychologists George Brown and Tirril Harris[2] found that depression is closely correlated with the number of bad things that have happened to you, especially if you had suffered a significant bereavement earlier in life, but there is no simple formula to explain depression and its severity. This leads us all to interpret the meaning of the events. Why was that particular event so upsetting and why did it have such a lasting impact?

This is where the cognitive approach comes in. Take memory. Talk to a depressed person about the past and what they say is dominated by negative occurrences. You (and they) have to work really hard to elicit a good-news story. They are not choosing to be morose, nor is it necessarily the effect of being depressed, although it becomes hard to separate cause and effect when thinking about mood and cognition. It turns out that in psychological research where recall is studied under controlled conditions, such as in response to a particular set of words or prompts, the depressed person is much more able to bring to mind negative associations than positive ones and does so more quickly. This is where the cognitive bias asserts itself. It's not that other items are forgotten but they are simply not at hand. The thoughts and memories that bubble up to the surface straight away are the negative ones. Imagine I ask the perfectly innocent question: what did you do last week? If you are depressed, your mind is flooded with all the bad, unpleasant, boring, frustrating, annoying things that happened, and this crowds out all the happy, pleasant, even banal and neutral things that happened. If you weren't depressed before, you certainly would be afterwards. It is easy to see why this becomes a vicious cycle. Starting off from a position of feeling low, further negative thoughts seem to be normal, the status quo, and low mood becomes self-sustaining.

Another characteristic that researchers like Mark Williams have discovered to be a feature of depressive thinking is over-generalisation, particularly of personal autobiographical memories.[3] Over-generalisation describes the difficulty people have, when depressed, in giving specific instances of behaviours, conversations and sequences, as well as in remembering one-off events in response to a question. Here's an example: tell me about school. They might say, "I hated it. I was bored; we all were," rather than, "I flunked my A levels but enjoyed the social side. In my last year I had a great group of friends." Or in response to a cue word, 'party': "Every birthday party I've ever hosted has been a disaster!" – instead of, for example, "I had my twenty-first at the local pub. It started well, but a few people had too much to drink and got into a fight. What a disaster!"

The over-generalised response leaves no room for reinterpretation or sparking off other memories that may put the event and its memory in context. It is like clicking on a link and being redirected. You find it hard to get out of this loop, which is now prompting only other similar globally negative thoughts with no prospect of resolution. In other words, you start to ruminate.

***

Eventually, I persuaded Thomas to come into hospital on the basis that he needed a break, he wouldn't have to stay long, we could change round his medication more quickly and, above all, he would be safe. Reluctantly, he agreed.

He was miserable. He hated the intrusion of constant observations, the lack of privacy and the general mess and chaos that pervades even the best psychiatric wards. Thomas was hard to get to know. He would describe his background as "dreary, boring, nothing ever happened... My mum and dad treated us well although there wasn't much show of affection. Church was a big thing. That really was the 'good news', but sometimes I almost wish there had been some kind of disaster; at least I'd have something to talk about."

A few weeks after adding in an additional powerful antidepressant, Thomas's mood started to lift and he was becoming more positive. His wife, Jan, visited and was pleased to see the improvement. He was bored and desperately missed the children. He implored me to allow him to go home. Again, this required negotiation and we agreed to a sequence of increasing periods of home leave, which were to be introduced gradually. We would work with him and his wife to gauge progress and adjust the leave accordingly. We weren't trying to make him a permanent resident in the hospital, but we also couldn't whip away all his support at once.

The first leave period of a few hours went well. We then agreed on a full day at home. He returned buoyed up and optimistic. In the ward round where Thomas spoke to other members of the team, nurses and ward psychologist, he seemed much better. He was fine about staying on the medication. He was not troubled by side effects and he had confidence that the treatment would work this time, as it had before. We discussed how, when he was discharged, we would need to talk to his employer. I would write whatever reports were necessary to say that the treatment was essential and there was no reason he couldn't continue his work. He was relieved; it would be a weight off his mind. Did he still feel guilty? Not at all. That was ridiculous; it was just the depression talking. Anyway, he'd had enough with all that religious nonsense. Jan said she would be happy to have him back home, even though he wasn't quite his normal self. We agreed on weekend leave. If that went well, the discharge date would be set for the following week.

That was the last time I saw Thomas. On the Tuesday, Jan came to the hospital to tell me what had happened. Tom had come home. He seemed calm. They had supper and went to bed. They made love; it was nice. The next morning he took the kids to school. After dropping them off, he must have gone straight to the nearby main road, parked and got out of his car. According to a bystander, he looked agitated and suddenly ran out in front of a lorry and was killed instantly.

They made love… a lorry… killed instantly…

I gasped for air.

Jan was unnaturally calm. She explained that she just had to 'keep it together' for the sake of the children. She didn't want to think about it. The nursing staff tried to comfort her but ended up being more comforted *by* her. She didn't blame anyone and was grateful for our help. The case would be sent to the coroner and she was worried about what effect the verdict might have on the family, for whom suicide was a grave sin. In the meantime, she was going to take the children to her mother's house.

Several weeks later, Jan phoned the ward. The coroner's verdict was accidental death. He knew Thomas was a voluntary patient on leave from a psychiatric ward and was suffering from depression, but there was no suicide note and he was obviously recovering, since he had been home for the weekend. Thomas hadn't spoken about suicide to anyone that day. They said that he might have been preoccupied and so didn't look where he was going. It was a busy main road. People get run over all the time.

Jan knew the other possible verdicts: suicide and an open verdict. I had thought the latter was the most likely. Researchers into suicide generally regard most open verdicts as really suicide, but things like the absence of a suicide note are influential. Accidental death seemed like a stretch, but we weren't going to argue. From the family's point of view, this was perhaps the best they could hope for amid such a tragedy. At least it avoided stigma.

***

Suicide was finally deemed legal in England and Wales in 1961, but it is still tainted by its criminal past.[4] Its decriminalisation came very late compared with the rest of Europe but was still ahead of Ireland, which only decriminalised attempted suicide in 1993. Many people still talk unwittingly of *committing* suicide, although 'taking one's own life' is the generally preferred terminology. Coroners' verdicts used to adopt the criminal standard of proof of 'beyond reasonable doubt', but following a High Court ruling in 2018, they can now judge 'on the balance of probabilities', the civil standard.

Nearly 1,800 people are killed on the roads in the UK each year. The numbers have been steadily falling since the Second World War but are perhaps levelling off now. From recent figures, about a quarter are pedestrians. This contrasts with around 6,000 deaths by suicide in the UK each year. Such rates have also tended to fall over the same period. In 2015 the age-standardised suicide rate for the UK was 16 per 100,000 for males and 5 per 100,000 for females. There are few reliable figures on the number of pedestrian or motor vehicle accidents that are in fact suicides.

It is a great challenge for us to understand suicide, let alone to prevent it. One approach is to try to get inside the mind of the individual who dies by suicide and, if you are a great writer, like Shakespeare or Tolstoy, put this at the centre of your drama; or if you are a psychologist, perform a psychological autopsy. Another approach is to view it from above, through large groups of people and trends over time. One person who could be said to have invented this approach was Émile Durkheim.[5]

Durkheim was born in 1858 in the French district of Lorraine into what would have been nine generations of rabbis had he not decided to take a different path. He published his monograph 'On Suicide' in 1897. The Industrial Revolution was well underway and societies in Europe were well ordered and monitored. From detailed and voluminous national statistics, Durkheim was able to observe suicide rates according to a huge array of variables: national, ethnic, economic, demographic, educational and what he called 'cosmic' (things like temperature and day length). He did so with a Talmudic attention to detail. He was also able to look at things like rates of insanity and alcoholism, but even with these it was the sociological perspective that he believed held the key.

Religion was the factor that caught his eye since, all else being equal, data from French cantons and German populations, stretching from Prussia to Austria to Bavaria, had striking differences in suicide rates between Protestants and Roman Catholics. There was a consistent excess in suicide rates in Protestants; in some regions there were three such deaths for every Catholic. Durkheim showed that the excess in Protestants pertained regardless of the base rate of suicide in any particular region and that it could not be accounted for by, for example, differing access to education. He argued that the precise rituals and doctrine didn't have much bearing either. In fact, it was the extent to which the religion, through its beliefs and practices, produces 'an intense collective life', which really mattered in inhibiting suicide. Protestantism, by its nature, was more individualistic and would not 'exercise the same moderating influence on suicide'. He discussed this in relation to what he called 'egotistical suicide'.

But what of non-believers? He writes:

To the extent that the believer has doubts…feels less solidarity with the religious faith to which he belongs, and frees himself from it, or to the extent that the individual becomes estranged from the family and the political community, he becomes a mystery to himself and then cannot escape the annoying and agonizing question: what is the point of it all?

This collective sense is vital, he explains, 'not because we need to sustain the illusion of some impossible immortality; it is because it is implicit in our moral being and cannot be lost'. If it is lost or collapses, 'the slightest cause for depression can give rise to desperate acts'. Furthermore:

> However individual a person may be, there is always something collective that remains… As for the inci-dents of private life that appear to be the immediate motive for suicide…they are in reality only incidental causes. If the individual gives way to the slightest adversity it is because the state of society has made him easy prey for suicide. (pp. 229–32)

Over a century after Durkheim, we still find ourselves oscil-lating between the individual and the collective in trying to unlock the causes of suicide. The same social factors (i.e. unem-ployment, divorce and recession) remain linked to higher suicide rates in the population. Curiously, war does not make suicide more likely. For all the suffering that follows in its wake, war induces a powerful common purpose which works against individuals taking their own lives. Other risk factors include being male, making a previous attempt, having a mental illness, being without hope, as well as drug and alcohol misuse. Modern clinical studies attempting to integrate these approaches have shown that having a religious affiliation may still attenuate the suicidal impulses in people suffering from depression.[6]

Is suicide common? It's all relative. Compared with road traffic accidents, the answer is yes. For a man in his late thirties, like Thomas, it is the commonest cause of death. But compared with depression, the answer is no; relative to that, suicide is exceedingly rare. Hence, there is difficulty in prediction. When looking back over cases of suicide, the vast majority belong to low- or only moderate-risk groups. This seems like a paradox but is a familiar pitfall of risk prediction. Because individual risk factors are not overwhelmingly strong, and because some of the risk factors themselves, such as depression, are common, it is a statistical inevitability that most people who die by suicide will come from a relatively large group of low-risk people. A greater but still minor proportion of people from a high-risk group (let's say men of a certain age with severe depression, alcohol dependence, who are chronically ill, widowed and unemployed) will take their own lives, but that subgroup will be numerically small in the wider scheme of things. The other problem is that the most reliable risk factors don't change: for example, being male. If you are a man, your risk is the same today as it was last year, and as it will be tomorrow.

***

I first had to come to terms with suicidal behaviour when I was a junior doctor working in an average-sized general hospital. For six months I was the first medic to deal with emergency admissions. The hospital had a very innovative approach to medical emergencies. They had several 'teams' dealing with particular emergencies so that expertise and experience could be built up and shared rapidly. There was a 'chest-pain team', a 'gastric-bleeding team' and another team for anyone over sixty-five years of age. It was striking how many people brought in by ambulance or turning up in Accident and Emergency (A&E) could be directed to one of a handful of teams. You'd have thought that a junior doctor left to deal with 'other' categories of emergency would have had very little to do – the occasional pneumonia or diabetic coma, perhaps. This was true except for one category which, in the 1980s, was massively increasing: deliberate self-poisoning by taking an overdose. It was not unusual for me to have to assess and admit to the medical ward ten such patients over the course of one night.

As a student I had seen how many such patients were treated. Taking an overdose of paracetamol can have deadly consequences through liver toxicity, and the older antidepressants can induce cardiac arrest, but many overdoses were less harmful benzodiazepines like Valium and Librium, or whatever else people had in their medicine cabinets: antibiotics, indigestion pills and so forth. Because of this relative lack of danger and the sheer number of cases that came after hours and at weekends, 'overdoses' were seen as a nuisance or, even worse, a group whose apparently self-inflicted condition deserved punishment. Some casualty staff delighted in carrying out the gastric lavage ('stomach pumping'), an extremely unpleasant procedure and not necessary in many cases; others insisted that the person have a urinary catheter – another unpleasant and often painful procedure seldom required, unless it is essential to monitor kidney function in someone who is very drowsy or in whom the drugs had blocked the passage of urine. Many staff were abrupt and unsympathetic. The culture was widespread if not universal. I shudder when I recall such behaviour and feel ashamed that I did nothing to intervene. I suppose I thought that it might actually be an effective deterrent – some people would be admitted time and again with the same sort of behaviour – and anyway, what did I know?

During these testing six months, I came to learn that being sympathetic and non-judgemental was actually the best strategy. I stress that this was not because I was exceptionally kind and understanding. It was, at that point, a matter of pragmatism. There were a lot of patients to get through. Some would need intensive medical resuscitation and you had to spot them early; others could cause havoc by being uncooperative and aggressive. The last thing you wanted to have to deal with on a busy night on-call was a person seeking to discharge themselves against medical advice and needing to be restrained as they ran out of the ward, or an entourage of angry and inebriated relatives demanding that you admit the person to the intensive care unit, or to the psychiatric hospital, or discharge them.

The overdose patients I saw were sometimes intoxicated, sometimes angry, sometimes indifferent. Most commonly, they were distressed young people who felt they were trapped and had run out of options. A simple, gentle, "tell me what happened" would invariably lead to a sorry tale of rejection, abuse or despair, the hurt of being dumped by a boyfriend or kicked out by your parents. At times the circumstances seemed genuinely intractable and the person at the centre was deeply troubled. Remaining brusque ("no need for all this drama, you'll be home in the morning") or didactic ("didn't you realise how dangerous paracetamol can be?") might have seemed justifiable but merely led to defiance and heightened distress.

One responsibility placed on the junior doctor or nurse specialist is to assess suicide risk or intent. Intuitively, the degree of planning, the steps taken to avoid being stopped or discovered, the lethality of the method (jumping in front of a train versus taking some tablets), must surely be important, although there is no simple formula for quantifying their cumulative effect. Simply asking the person why they did it is worth a try but rarely elicits a useful answer. An empathic, unhurried encounter will be rewarded with a thoughtful response, but even if given in good faith, it cannot always be taken at face value. People rarely say that they did it to make their partner feel guilty, or so that their landlord wouldn't chuck them out, even though such explanations fit well with the circumstances leading up to the episodes. While many would say, "I just wanted to die" or "I'd had enough, there's nothing to live for," my impression was that, after a degree of trust had been established, the majority really felt more ambiv-alent: "I don't really know why I did it"; "I was confused, overwhelmed"; "I just wanted the way I was feeling to end." These explanations rang true to me.

Psychiatrists have sought to distinguish self-harm from suicide. The term 'parasuicide' was proposed to emphasise the distinction but has not really stood the test of time. The epidemiology of the two does show that they tend to affect different groups. Self-harm is much more common: about 400–500 per 100,000 people each year. It tends to occur in young people and declines with age. Suicide shows no such decline. Parasuicide is more common in women; suicide in men. However, there is plenty of overlap. Louis Appleby is the director of the National Confidential Inquiry into Suicide and Homicide by People with Mental Illness (NCISH) and he has come up with the 'rule of 50', a useful and salutary mnemonic: 50% of people who die by suicide have a history of self-harm; risk of suicide may be increased fiftyfold in the year following self-harm; and 1 in 50 people seen in A&E after self-harm will be dead a year later. Self-harm lights a fuse which, as it meanders, will usually fizzle out; but every so often, it evades being extinguished and ends fatally. The NCISH has also highlighted the immediate period after discharge from hospital as being a particularly high-risk period for suicide, especially the first week and indeed the first day, as it turned out to be so fatefully for Thomas.

***

My attempt to deal with Thomas's death and the sense that I had failed him and his family did, I think, drive me into the research literature in search of solace and, perhaps, as a way of avoiding the raw pain of the experience. It was there that I discovered some fascinating insights into suicide at the population level. The big-picture, epidemiological perspective may, to some researchers, seem to be as dry, impersonal and cold as the archives of accumulated death certificates which support it. But it is the changes brought about at the population level which have made a difference.

Some of these changes have been fortuitous. When carbon-monoxide-containing coal gas began to be substituted by natural gas in the 1950s, a rising tide of death was halted and reversed, especially among women, for whom gassing was the most common method of suicide. (Think of the poet Sylvia Plath, who died in her London terrace by putting her head inside a gas oven in 1963.) This simple change in fuel led to a dramatic decrease in overall suicide rates. What epidemiologists noticed to their surprise was the lack of 'method substitution': when this method was cut off, people did not necessarily search deliberately for an alternative.

Looking at trends over time, it can be seen that later, suicide by inhaling car exhaust did start to creep up, especially in men, but this too was curtailed by legislation introducing catalytic converters in 1993.[7] A more planned and deliberate 'means restriction' intervention was to reduce the number of tablets of paracetamol and other analgesics that could be purchased at one go. Again it took a change in the law in 1998 to do this, but it led to a fall in mortality with little evidence for substitution. All of the successful suicide-prevention strategies we have discovered have been tactical and simple, almost embarrassingly so.

I remember watching a stand-up comedian whose routine went something like this:

> The government really cares about us, y'know? Like, once my mate was feeling really depressed and thought – enough – I'm gonna top myself. So he goes down to the chemists to buy some paracetamol and guess what, it only comes in packs of sixteen! I mean, come on, do they really think that's gonna stop someone who's suicidal? Like we can't work out that all we need to do is come back tomorrow? Maybe that's why it's 'commit suicide' because you've really got to, like, commit.

But common sense can only take you so far. When psychiatrist Keith Hawton and colleagues wrote their report, they worked out that over about eleven years, 765 fewer people had died thanks to the tablet-packaging legislation in England and Wales alone.[8] Paracetamol overdose remains common, but less fatal, thanks to this humble alteration. Add to that other simple changes, like removing potential ligature points from which a person might try to hang themselves in psychiatric wards; putting barriers around train-station platforms and high walkways. In South Asia, the authorities should make organophosphate pesticides a little less easy to get hold of, and in the US, if only they would further restrict gun ownership – all this would reduce suicide rates markedly. It seems that despite the weight of history, of societal pressures and the ravages of mental illness, after all the Hamlet-like deliberation and Karenina-like inevitability, the final act can be a deadly yet fleeting impulse, one weak enough to succumb to a momentary distraction or a trivial barrier.

And yet some of the people I speak to have been remarkably determined to take their own life. They might have long histories of mental illness and multiple attempts. I remember one man who had come through a paracetamol overdose, meticulously planned and executed – no impulsive act this – leading to near liver failure from which he eventually recovered. He told me of his fantasy that after his suicide, he would somehow be able to observe the scene, as if from the heavens, of his family gathered round his grave in mourning: his wife admonishing herself for her lack of affection; the teenage children weeping inconsolably, wishing they could have had more time with their father; the work boss, once so disdainful, now broken, begging for forgiveness; the wider world, paying tribute to a wonderful humanitarian, sadly unappreciated in his lifetime, who would be sorely missed. It was a brave admission. I also remember listening to a distraught woman whose own father had died by suicide. She was desperate to rid from her mind thoughts of going down the same route, saying she could never do that to her children, and me feeling reassured. I wrote in my notes that while a suicide risk, she had 'protective factors'. She did, however, take her own life. Such narratives cannot be resolved. There is an idea, even in the minds of some mental health professionals, that suicide is a selfish act. But it is hard to imagine what it must be like to believe you are so awful, so toxic that even your bereaved children would feel they are better off without you.

***

What might Thomas have been thinking when, as it appears, he was planning his last twenty-four hours? The man who 'thinks too much' seemed to have been living in the moment. One can't help speculating that, having decided he was going to take his own life, he experienced a profound sense of calm. His relinquishing of 'all that religious nonsense' did not leave him yearning for some other source of consolation; nor was it a satisfying resolution to doubt in the supernatural. He had not, patently, come to his senses as I allowed myself, in my rationalist bubble, to think at the time. It was, or so I surmise, an utter transformation of his world, his 'moral being' as Durkheim would have it. It was at this point that he, as a social creature, ceased to exist.

In hindsight, the loss of religion should have been a red flag. But why could he not see a way out, an alternative? Perhaps this goes back to the over-generalised memory that he, like many people with depression, exhibited from the beginning. Psychologists have shown that thinking of the past in this non-specific, generic way makes it hard for us to re-evaluate the past and its personal significance.[9] And what this does, crucially, is prevent us from learning new lessons from it; it limits creative thinking. So when your world collapses and you can see no prospect of inventing another, there is indeed no future, no hope and nothing to live for. But to look at our past and see how many different people we have already been – that is the key to imagining a future we want to live in: what might happen, where I'd like to be, how my life could be different.[10]

4

Just the Two of Us

The fast bleep brought a jolt of alertness to the early-evening calm. An emergency. I was the Inside Duty Doctor, covering the hospital for urgent calls. 'Violent incident on the locked ward'. That was my ward. I knew immediately who would be at the centre of it. It had to be Junior.

When I arrived, slightly out of breath with my keys jangling, there was a standoff. Junior had repeatedly asked to leave – he just wanted a bit of space away from everyone, somewhere to play his guitar – but had not been allowed. He was deemed too volatile and unpredictable.

He was an intimidating presence: six foot plus, shaved head and probably sixteen stone of muscle. A struggle ensued. He was waving his guitar at the staff who were lining up in a semi-circle in front of the door blocking his path. The charge nurse, a man in his late forties, was trying to 'de-escalate' the situation; speaking softly, trying to placate. He had a good relationship with Junior. They both had family connections in Jamaica and liked to talk about home.

"C'mon, Junior. Put your guitar down. This isn't going to work. You know you are on a Section and can only go out accompanied. Perhaps we'll go for a walk in the grounds a bit later. Why don't we go to your room?"

The rest of the staff nodded.

"Let's talk about this," I added. "We were going to review the Section soon, but you need to calm down."

"Uncle Tom and his merry men," he sneered, fixing the charge nurse in a stare. "How does it feel to be a descendant of slaves turned slave owner?" Then, turning to me, he laughed joylessly. "Let my people go!"

He raised the guitar, holding it by the neck, trembling with rage. We shrank away.

"Put it down," the charge nurse said firmly.

"OK, OK, I'll put it down; don't get your knickers in a twist," he said mockingly.

He placed the guitar carefully on the floor. It was a beautiful instrument, a finely polished Spanish acoustic, inlaid with mother of pearl. "Let's retire to the drawing room. And boy, bring me a glass of your finest Chateau Haloperidol!"

The tension subsided. We eased back. He stood over the guitar, looking at it wistfully. Then suddenly he raised his foot and stamped down hard, cracking the soundboard. He turned around to face the wall with his arms raised in a pose of mock surrender. Two nurses took hold of him on either side and he was escorted to the 'time out' area.

It was a shocking moment. It brought to mind a scene in the 1973 Robert Altman film *The Long Goodbye*, a reworking of the Raymond Chandler classic. Private detective Philip Marlowe is meeting the gangster Marty Augustine who, in an unusual twist, is portrayed as Jewish rather than Italian-American.

Someone owes him money. He's not happy. He turns towards his girlfriend and caresses her, extolling her beauty. Out of the blue he smashes a Coke bottle against her face in a sickening act of brutality. He turns towards Marlowe and says, "That's someone I love. You, I don't even like."

Junior had a diagnosis of manic depression, or bipolar disorder as it is now called. He was in his late twenties. The son of a professional musician who was well known in Jamaica, he too was musical, an accomplished guitarist and songwriter. Brought up in the UK, he excelled academically and studied law at a prestigious university before succumbing to his first illness. He was also an expert in martial arts (or so he said).

***

Many people suffer from mood or affective disorders as psychiatrists call them. Those who suffer from depression may have distinct bouts which recur but with periods of normal mood (euthymia) in between. Occasionally they have episodes of elevated mood. When extreme this is called mania, which implies a break from reality in which mood drives delusions and hallucinations – for example, the belief that one is fabulously wealthy, in possession of special powers, a genius or superhero; or hearing heavenly choirs, the music of the spheres or the voice of God. The person with mania has boundless energy and may go without sleep for days on end, eventually grinding to a halt through sheer exhaustion. Speech may be so sped up as to be incomprehensible.

More often the episodes are mild and short-lived: 'hypomania', a potentially confusing term that just means an elevated
mood short of mania. Hypomania is sometimes the result of
antidepressant treatment acting on an over-sensitive biological mood-control system. A person with hypomania is also full
of energy. Initially it's infectious, but it soon becomes wearing.
Their speech may be fast and furious but you *can* follow it
(barely). They are optimistic without being irrational, but
their judgement and priorities are distorted and relationships
tend to become strained by the person's self-absorption and
lack of consideration for others.

Oddly, the person with mania and indeed hypomania is
rarely happy. Sadness and happiness are normally the poles of
a person's mood. Just as depression takes the person beyond
the familiar landscape of sadness into an altogether darker,
bleaker place, hypomania and mania go outside the normal
bounds of happiness to a place where nothing is constant and
change is fast. It is an impatient world where no one suffers
fools. *I want it and I want it now*, mania seems to say. It's less
like happiness and more like irritability, a poorly understood
emotional state at the heart of many interpersonal and psychiatric difficulties.[1] The person with hypomania may start out
positive and generous – they may give away their money and
possessions, and their affections – but they soon feel unsatis-
fied when the world does not reciprocate. It's too damn slow;
people are idiots! Generosity may lead to penury and new
schemes go pear-shaped. All this is frustrating for the person
suffering from hypomania, and such frustration can lead to
aggression and even violence.

Just as there may be a biological mood-control system that senses chemical disruption – be it antidepressants, alcohol or stimulants – it seems natural to infer a psychological regulator which is always trying to keep our mood within reasonable bounds. Once mood runs outside the range, it becomes unstable, wobbly or labile. The person with mania can suddenly flip into maudlin despair and then back to ecstasy, leaving bystanders drained and uncomprehending. A skilled psychiatrist can try to make use of this phenomenon to impose some measure of control over the person with mania by introducing a note of melancholy. Suddenly the patient stops and becomes reflective. It doesn't last long, but it's often long enough to snatch a short, meaningful conversation about the mess they are in.

People often wonder what it might be like to turn the dial up a little higher than normal. Haven't we all had times when we were on a roll and everything just *flowed*? Anything we wanted to say came out right; we were witty, clever, erudite. Our movements were fluid and graceful, our senses heightened. People sometimes describe periods of great creativity and energy, possibly balanced by periods in the doldrums when quiet contemplation takes over. The psychiatric term is 'cyclothymia'. If the old trope of madness and creativity has any credence at all, it is probably related to this kind of controlled bipolarity. And maybe you can't really experience joy without having gone through despair.

Where does the bipolarity come from, this cycling up and down? It is too easy to see one as a natural consequence of the other. Hence, there are notions of 'flight into mania', as if, having suffered depression for so long, it is possible simply to catapult out of it, up and beyond. More appealing and also more credible is the notion that after a period of mania or hypomania, when the individual is surrounded by the destruction wrought by their condition, depression is inevitable. Whether that is an adequate explanation is moot. It is certainly a recognised pattern.

The aptly named Swiss psychiatrist Jules Angst and co-workers have followed up large numbers of people with bipolar disorder over many decades. They have found that those whose bipolar disorder is severe enough to require hospitalisation can end up spending a fifth of their lives in an episode, having regular, recurrent swings in mood. On average, each episode lasts about three months and occurs very roughly 0.4 times per year.[2] Usually there is a period of euthymia in between, but this can be fleeting, sometimes a matter of a few hours of calm, before one kind of storm or another. Many experts believe that this pattern is inherited, hard wired by a genetic defect, but that is yet to be established.

Sometimes the regularity is uncanny. Such rhythmicity is seen in biological systems throughout nature. Many mammals undergo well-timed hibernation and some, including primates, have oestrus cycles when they are 'on heat'. Reproductive cycles are of course part of human female physiology, but it's hard to discern a related behavioural cycle. Cases of regular manic-depressive cycles around a twenty-eight-day period have been recorded, although it's worth saying that one particularly noteworthy case, published in the *British Medical Journal* in 1959 by biological psychiatrist John Crammer, described a forty-eight-year-old *man*.[3]

Many of our cycles are circadian, that is, we sleep and wake in time with the sun. Such cycles are underpinned by a complex system of hormonal and neurophysiological controls. Disruption to such cycles, as in shift work or jet lag, can have profound effects on our well-being and mood. Such imposed shifts in phase are known to trigger bipolar episodes in those with a vulnerability. For instance, it seems that flying from the US to the UK is particularly liable to induce a hypomanic episode, but not in the other direction.[4]

***

It wasn't feasible to speak to Junior that night. The atmosphere on the ward was tense. He accepted, after some prevarication, the extra dose of haloperidol, which is a powerful sedative and antipsychotic; after all, it was his idea.

The next morning, I returned to the ward for routine duties. The staff reported that at about 3 a.m. Junior had drifted into a light sleep. Now, he was up and about and yes, irritable, making snide remarks and puns about hitting the high notes, how "the joint was jumpin' last night 'round midnight" and so on. He was also causing problems by egging on other patients, most of whom were more chaotic and disturbed than him, and certainly less articulate. "You have nothing to lose but your chains," he'd say to them. "Let's make a bid for freedom tonight, jailbirds!" "*One flew east, one flew west, one flew over the cuckoo's nest*. Ha!"

I popped my head round his door. "Can I come in?"

"Can't stop you. I have no rights. I'm the colony, the township, the occupied territory," he said with a snarl, switching from Indian, to South African to Arabic accents.

I noticed his guitar, leaning against his bed, forlorn. The damage didn't look too bad, considering.

"Shame about the…"

"Yeah, I'm an idiot… *While my guitar gently weeps…*" he murmured, half-heartedly breaking into song.

We discussed 'being on a Section', how last night would be viewed as a setback. I understood his frustration. He really was improving. We had decided not to stop his accompanied leave (with a member of staff) but that he did have to wait until there was someone free before he could go out for half an hour or so. He needed to be patient. This was a locked ward, but it was not a secure unit and no, it was not a prison. A certain degree of cooperation was required. We had to work together. He was back on the lithium, the first mood-stabilising drug to be discovered and undoubtedly effective. It seemed to have helped. He'd been fine for over a year, the longest spell since he first became ill, until he stopped taking it.

He had been in hospital for at least two months now. He was brought in by the police, having been reported hanging around Westminster Bridge. It wasn't clear if he had been contemplating jumping into the Thames or heading towards Parliament. When approached by police, he was apparently 'talking gibberish' about starting another riot (there had been riots in Brixton not long before). Rather than arresting him, they took him to hospital.

Did he agree to go along with the regime? He was looking bored already and getting restless. One thing about people who are hypomanic is that they notice everything about you and will home in on any blemish or spot, any unfortunate choice of words, any perceived weakness, and exploit it.

"You like this, don't you?" he said accusingly. I looked blankly back at him. "The control, the power, the oppressive *regime*."

"No, actually, I hate it."

Junior was contemptuous. Why, then, was the ward full of black men?

He had a point. It was true in that the number of black patients in psychiatric hospitals was much higher than would be expected, even in areas of London with high numbers of black and ethnic minority groups. It was a topic of concern and some good research.[5] Was it something to do with susceptibility to childhood or even intrauterine infections in immigrants from the Caribbean and Africa – who lack previous exposure and hence immunity to common viruses – somehow affecting brain development or functioning? (Difficult to prove, as it may be too subtle to show up on brain scans.) Was it genetic? (Unlikely, as there didn't seem to be much history of the illness in their families.) Was it to do with migration? (Could be, although most of the patients were second or third generation.) Was it due to cannabis or other drug use? (Possible, although the use of cannabis is equally high among white and black youth.) Was it due to labelling, that is, people with different cultural attitudes being given a psychiatric diagnosis through lack of understanding, and yes, perhaps an effort to control? (Unlikely, since Jamaican psychiatrists working in London made the same diagnoses.) Or was it simply a reaction to racism endemic in society? I was prepared to accept that society was racist but maintained that I and my profession were not. Most people I worked with held liberal values. We enjoyed diversity. We were just picking up the pieces.

As for labelling, colleagues and I researched this formally using case vignettes. We asked two hundred or so practising British psychiatrists to comment on the likely diagnosis and whether they would anticipate problems, such as violence, if the case were real.[6] Secretly, we altered the ethnicity of the vignette to see if this influenced responses. We found that diagnostic labelling was subtly influenced by whether the person in the vignette was Afro-Caribbean or white, but more strikingly, if the person was black and male, the risk of violence was perceived to be somewhat greater. We discussed this in terms of 'race thinking', a sociological concept which sees stereotyping as pervasive and usually (but not always) nega- tive. Fortunately, if brought to people's attention, it can be counteracted, unlike ideological racism. It was thought, there- fore, that calling professional people out as 'racist' may be necessary but often led only to defensive denial and counter- accusations. This was some years before the McPherson Report on the police's handling of the Stephen Lawrence case and the concept of institutional racism.[7]

However, at that moment, standing in Junior's room, I took the bait. Of course I wasn't a racist. I had noticed he was always going on about it, making unfair inferences. He was simply not taking responsibility for his actions was my summation.

"You *would* say that, wouldn't you? The white man doesn't even realise he is being racist when he talks to the black man. Just as the black man doesn't realise that he can never be himself in a white man's culture." Now getting heated: "You know nothing. *A man's a man for aw that*, Rabbie Burns, Rabbi Sigmund… I am a better psychiatrist than you'll ever be!" Now shouting: "Go and read Frantz Fanon and then you can talk to me!"

***

Frantz Fanon, I learned, was born in 1925 in Martinique, then a French Caribbean colony. He was the son of a middle-class black father and a mixed-race mother. He fought with the Free French Forces during the Second World War in North Africa and France, where he was wounded and awarded the *Croix de Guerre*. After the war, he studied medicine in Lyon, specialising in psychiatry. As part of his qualifications he submitted a treatise that was to become his first book, *Black Skin, White Masks*,[8] which I found in the library. Apparently, the university rejected his thesis as 'inappropriately subjective' and, in 1952, he submitted instead a case study on a more mainstream neuropsychiatric topic.[9]

His first major appointment in 1953 was to the staff of the Blida-Joinville psychiatric hospital in Algeria with eight psychiatrists in charge of 2,500 beds. He instituted many reforms, brought in occupational therapy and encouraged patients to participate in the governance of the hospital. He tried to integrate European and African patients but found that while beneficial to the former, the latter became 'apathetic and hostile'. He attributed this to his mistaken adoption of a 'colonial policy of assimilation', which he corrected by bringing in indigenous healing practices.[10]

In *Black Skin, White Masks*, Fanon draws on literature, anthropology and psychoanalysts like Freud, Adler and Jung, as well as philosophers such as Jean-Paul Sartre and Hegel. He talks about the white man's fear of the black man (which he called 'Negrophobia', though this term is now antiquated), based on sexual jealousy, as well as describing how his own and his ancestral experience of racism is internalised, leading to unresolvable conflict. 'The Antillean is a slave to his cultural imposition. After having been a slave of the white man, he enslaves himself'.[11] In 1956 he joined the Algerian *Front de Libération Nationale* (FLN), taking a more active revolutionary position against French neocolonialism. He died of leukaemia in 1961 while serving as an emissary for Algeria in Ghana.

I should have known about Fanon and could see why he was an inspiration to psychiatric patients of Caribbean heritage. The concept of race thinking might have chimed with Frantz Fanon in the earlier phases of his theorising around *Black Skin, White Masks*, but not when he became more radical.

***

Junior's irritability and grandiosity were subsiding. It was becoming possible to have longer conversations with him without flitting from topic to topic (sometimes called 'flight of ideas') and without the wearing confrontational banter. There were important matters to discuss: salvaging a career, patching up fractured relations with friends and family, avoiding psychiatric hospitals in the future. The tone was sober, even melancholy. I wondered whether he was becoming depressed or whether, as others who knew him better believed, this was what he was really like: a thoughtful, contemplative, pensive young man. There was still the occasional barb at my white privilege: "That's easy for you to say" and "I bet you never had to struggle." We also had some non-clinical chats about music. I told him I played piano a little. We both enjoyed jazz.

Accompanied leave, a part of the terms of his being detained in hospital under a section of the Mental Health Act, was still a source of conflict and frustration. Junior understood the principle that if he went off on his own while unwell, he might get into trouble and that the restriction was gradually being lifted. But for him the pace was too slow. I was a trainee psychiatrist at the time, so decisions around sections were not mine but those of the consultant. I had an idea to relieve the boredom and build on our improving rapport: I said I would take him on his next accompanied leave within the hospital grounds and he should bring the guitar.

Off we went, to the hospital gym. At one end, there was a disused stage, covered in dust, loaded with broken gym equipment, a table-tennis table, empty filing cabinets and other bits of junk. But there, under a green canvas cover, was a full-sized Blüthner concert grand piano, the same kind Paul McCartney used on 'Let It Be'. I knew it was playable, having used it for the hospital Christmas panto. Junior was transfixed and could only say, "Wow." This was the piano that virtuoso John Ogdon had played when he was a patient here a few years earlier.[12] His serious mental illness, perhaps a variant of manic depression, was well publicised, and during one spell he had used the hospital as a base while performing concerts in central London.

"So, let's have a jam," Junior said, pulling up a chair and tuning his cracked but otherwise functioning instrument. Amateur musicians will be familiar with the situation in which those gathered throw out names of songs and artists, hoping to find some common ground. It can be disappointing. What about some standards, I suggested. How about Gershwin's 'Summertime'?[13] That never fails.

A few rounds of that and we were nicely warmed up. Junior knew the words. The music flowed and we both relaxed. The setting was so different from our usual one and we both had the feeling that we were in cahoots, bunking off.

"George Gershwin – *Porgy and Bess* – how come you have this young Jewish guy from Brooklyn taking on the deepest, darkest most profound Negro experience?" he asked.

"Isn't it a mark of his genius that the music is universal?"

"Good tunes, I agree, but talk about cultural appropriation. You Jews have got your own dark history, so why take ours?"

I didn't want to spoil the ambience, but where was he going with this? Suddenly it made sense. All that stuff about 'let my people go', occupied territories, Rabbie Burns, Rabbi Sigmund… It wasn't just a play on the idea of Jews as victims turned aggressors (and my Scottish accent), it was aimed at me personally. This was his attempt to find some vulnerability that he might exploit, perhaps to restore the power imbalance between us as he saw it. He had decided I must be Jewish. I wasn't going to get into a discussion about my background or private life. Such boundaries should be preserved to maintain professional distance. You can be friendly, but in the end, you can't be a friend. I tried to change the subject.

"Right, how about a twelve-bar blues?" I crashed out a few chords and we got going.

"*Can the blue man sing the whites or are they hypo-crites to sing the blues,*" he crooned with gusto as we ended on a flamboyant major seventh.

"Let's dial it down a little. How about some smooth jazz?" I suggested.

We swapped a few names. I suggested a Grover Washington Jr hit – it has a tricky chromatically descending intro, but after that there's a simple riff you can improvise around.

"Nice!" said Junior. "It's one of my seduction tunes, for the more mature lady."

Just the two of us...[14]

We chuckled; ambience restored.

I looked at my watch. We had been off the ward for over an hour. I thought about how powerful music was at connecting people and reaching those parts that no drugs or even words could reach. But it was time to get back. I closed the lid on the piano, Junior gathered up his guitar. Running his hand over the body, he winced.

"I think it's repairable – hope so."

I nodded reassuringly.

"Oh, and thanks for that," he said softly and sincerely. "It was fun."

"Yeah, it was."

He suddenly stopped as we were leaving. "So, are you Jewish?"

I hesitated. "Yes."

He looked me in the eye. "By the way, I'm black."

5

You Are What You Eat

Has there ever been a more catchy, more nonsensical slogan than 'you are what you eat'? In contrast, 'eat to live, don't live to eat' is sensible but hardly gets the juices flowing. Hunger and the drive to eat is one of our most powerful biological drives. However, as with the sexual drive, it is the vast web of culture – made up of ritual, mores, commercialisation and ethics – that now governs our eating behaviour rather than the simple evolutionary imperatives.

Turkey Christmas dinner with all the trimmings. Sleek modernist foodie temples serving up foam, edible flowers and slimy offal on a rectangular slate. Raw fish carved as exquisitely as jewellery. Rotting milk curd becoming a thousand cheeses. Red-hot reptilian Asian street food. Genetically modified tofu. Deep-fried cod and chips wrapped in yesterday's news in a faded seaside town. A trillion identical hamburgers. Takeaway curry on Friday night. The condemned prisoner's last meal. The body and blood. Fasts and feasts. Chicken soup with magical healing properties.

The control of appetite is managed by a complex but beautifully balanced neural–humeral programme. This is part of what physiologists call homeostasis, the ability of the body to control its internal environment so that it always has enough energy. Lack of food prompts the release of hormones ('humours') such as cholecystokinin and ghrelin,[1] which are orexigenic (*orexis* is Greek for appetite) – we get hungry and seek food. As that food hits the stomach, it causes the release of hormones such as insulin and leptin, chemical messengers which tell the brain's engine room, the hypothalamus, to stop eating (anorexigenic) – leading us to feel full.

Not only are there many other hormones running through the bloodstream, there are also electrical messages to be conveyed through the nervous system. The main electrical cable connecting the gut and the brain is the vagus nerve. The stomach sends electrical signals up into the brain to make us hungry or full, as well as triggering reflex behaviours ranging from the basic (e.g. salivation) to the highly complex (booking a table at Escoffier's). A group of cells called 'agouti-related peptide-expressing neurones' in the hypothalamus seem to be key to this process. Experiments on rats in the 1950s showed that lesions to the lateral hypothalamus could halt feeding behaviour, while electrical stimulation could keep it going indefinitely. It's too simplistic to call it an 'on-and-off' switch, but the role of the hypothalamus is undisputed.[2]

Brain activity fans out from the hypothalamus – which sits at the top of the brain stem, underneath the thalamus, the brain's sensory relay station – upwards to regions in the mid-brain underlying motivation and reward, producing in us feelings of liking and desire. From there, the activity continues on to higher executive control regions in the cortex where we can mull over such sensations (i.e. plan when to repeat them, or feel guilty and contemplate going on a diet). Notice, when it comes to food, how soon homeostasis and physiological balance slips into notions of moral balance. Take this process and throw it into the real world and you can end up with a standoff: homeostatic eating versus hedonic eating (eating for pleasure). Even some hard-nosed neuroscientists cannot resist this conflict analogy.[3]

Anorexia nervosa, literally, is loss of appetite due to a nervous or mental condition as opposed to a physical condition such as cancer or chronic infection. The term was coined in 1873 by Sir William Gull as affecting 'mostly young women', but the symptoms have been traced back to antiquity.[4] Many patients and clinicians do not regard the loss of appetite as central to the disorder, which instead is characterised by an intense fear of gaining weight and of being fat, and a corresponding desire to be thin. This leads either to food restriction or to bingeing and purging. Some patients, usually in retrospect, will say that they did not lose their appetite – far from it, they endured constant hunger – but, like the character in Kafka's short story 'A Hunger Artist', it was their determination and virtuoso ability to control those feelings that marked them out. Others observe that after a while, the desire to eat lessens, perhaps masked by the dull nausea that accompanies starvation. This is due to the body breaking down its own reserves of fat, producing chemical by-products, ketones, which circulate in the blood, suppressing appetite and giving the breath a characteristic sweet-sickly smell.

In Gull's London, tuberculosis was endemic and would have been the first condition to spring to a doctor's mind if asked to see a young person who had lost a lot of weight. Anorexia nervosa was therefore something of a medical curiosity and part of the 'differential diagnosis' of tuberculosis. It was only in the 1950s that the disorder started to become more noticed and probably more prevalent. This time round it came with some heavy emotional baggage. Psychoanalysts like Hilde Bruch explicated the core psychological elements such as the difficulty a girl may have navigating the transition into womanhood, into becoming a separate sexual being apart from her family, and the underlying disorder of body image.[5] In the 1970s, feminist thinkers like Susie Orbach added their perspectives and started to critique aspects of eating, dieting and being fat in contemporary life.[6]

This picture of anorexia nervosa is very familiar.[7] We've all read in magazines or seen on TV the heartrending accounts of adolescent girls terrified of being fat. We know where it goes: self-starvation, family anguish and sometimes premature death. Body image is often illustrated cleverly by showing a thin young woman looking into a mirror and seeing reflected back her overweight doppelgänger.

***

Caitlín was different. She had been referred to me with the label '?atypical eating disorder'. She had just turned forty for one thing, and she didn't think she was fat. On the contrary, she agreed that she was on the thin side, although she tended to underplay and perhaps underestimate how pale and scrawny she looked. She hadn't had a period in years. Her problem was that she had lost her appetite. The doctors referring her had suspected an 'organic' or brain problem – perhaps a tumour of the pituitary gland, which could account for amenorrhoea (lack of menstruation), or of the hypothalamus causing a reduction in appetite.[8] But a normal MRI scan soon put paid to these possibilities. I was intrigued and decided to find out more about her symptoms, especially her 'loss of appetite'. She didn't seem much interested in the conversation.

"People make such a fuss about food. 'What would you like to eat?' 'Shall we go out for a meal?' 'Isn't that yummy!' 'Tastes delicious'. On and on they go. I can't be bothered with it."

Her diet comprised crispbread with lettuce, black tea and sometimes an apple. It wasn't just that she didn't enjoy food; she didn't think she should and wasn't sure that anyone should.

"It's just a biological function. I can't stand it when people, women usually, go on about having 'a complex relationship with food'. How can you have a relationship with, with…a doughnut? There are so many more important things to worry about."

Caitlín spoke in bursts followed by long silences. She often looked preoccupied and distracted.

"What sort of things?" I asked after a pause.

"What? Sorry, I was miles away."

"You said there were more important things to worry about. What sort of things?"

"Oh, you know…"

That exchange with Caitlín seemed to sum her up. Nothing substantial went into her mouth and nothing much came out of it. Her philosophy was that food was there to keep us alive

– why did it have to be pleasurable? And she had that attitude about everything.

Caitlín was brought up on a small farm in Ireland. She was the youngest of four; the only girl. Her father died suddenly of a heart attack when she was in her late teens. Her mother had worked on the farm and raised the children. The two older brothers ran the farm. The younger one had begun to train as a priest but had changed his mind and become a social worker. Caitlín did well at school and left home to go to a UK university to study history. She felt bad about leaving her mother whom she loved dearly. Her mum was a great cook, warm and giving, but at that time seemed to be in a state of constant numbness following the loss of her husband. Her mother had become 'clingy' in a way that Caitlín found stifling, and she felt she had to get away. Life had been hard on the farm with not much money around. Caitlín was suited to academia and took with her an earnestness beyond her years, frugality and self-sufficiency.

Was she just depressed? It is not difficult to see how low mood dulls all pleasurable feelings; that's why a core symptom of depression is anhedonia (literally lack of pleasure). It's less common, but some people find that low mood leads to 'comfort eating', in which the aim may be to chase the vanishing opportunities for pleasurable sensations, but the result is usually more despair and self-loathing.

I asked the standard questions about mood:

- How did she see the future? "The future will happen regardless of what I think."

- Did she think her life was worth living? "At the moment, yes. I have work to do."
- Did she feel guilty about anything? "Yes, lots of things."
- Did she think she was a good person? "Depends what you mean by 'good.'"
- Did she think she was depressed? "Mmm, not sure. Possibly."

All answers were delivered with the minimum elaboration. It was not that she seemed deliberately evasive, but I got the sense that Caitlín was someone who sought to be out of reach, to create as little impression as possible. She didn't show conventional signs of being depressed but was going to be hard to pigeonhole (like most of my patients).

I soldiered on: "You wouldn't say you were happy, then?"

"No, I definitely wouldn't. Not because I'm depressed, whatever that is. I don't expect to be happy, unlike most people these days. Historically, we have no right to be. Happiness is next to…emptiness. Live your life, try to do good or at least don't cause harm. That's enough for me."

I mentioned medication, antidepressants, not because I was convinced they would be useful at the moment, but just to find out where we stood on the subject. Happy pills? No way. After a few minutes of silence, I changed tack.

"How do you see yourself, as in, your body?"

"What do you mean?"

"Do you like yourself, the way you look?"

After a long, thoughtful pause, she answered, "I'm not sure they are the same thing."

She was right about that, but that was a whole new discussion and we had run out of time.

It was going to take a while to get to know Caitlín. After my first encounter with her, an assessment taking about an hour and a half, I suggested she come back in a month's time. I was not offering her psychotherapy with a set number of regular sessions every week or fortnight, or psychoanalysis which might be even more frequent and open-ended (and for which I have not been trained). This was a regular NHS outpatient clinic in a general hospital. Still, I felt I had to offer *something*.

I suggested maybe she put a bit of cream cheese on the crispbread. She said OK, she would try that.

***

What is body image? Sigmund Freud famously said:

> The ego is first and foremost a bodily ego; it is not merely a surface entity, but is itself the projection of a surface. If we wish to find an anatomical analogy for it we can best identify it with the 'cortical homunculus' of the anatomists, which stands on its head in the cortex, sticks up its heels, faces backwards and, as we know, has its speech-area on the left-hand side. The notion of an inner sense, or picture or three-dimensional model of the body in the mind being built upon but ultimately different from the physical body is a powerful one.[9]

Writing in the 1920s, Freud was drawing on contemporary thinking in neurology, where the concept of the body *schema*, a perfect little map of the body that lived inside the brain, was taking hold. That the map was a representation rather than a strict copy to scale became clear early in the twentieth century and was elaborated with the introduction of 'body image', a term attributed to Paul Schilder, a neuropsychiatrist and former pupil of Freud, in 1935.

Neurologists noted that damage to the parietal lobe on the right[10] could result in some very strange syndromes affecting bodily sensations, particularly on the left side of the body. In some instances the person seemed to be cut in half, ignoring or disowning their left side entirely. This syndrome, referred to as neglect or hemi-neglect, is a phenomenon well recognised today but still only partially understood. What stands out, though, is the lateralisation: the hallmark of neurological disorders of body image is that they are almost invariably asymmetrical, usually affecting the limbs on the left side.

But there is another aspect of body schema which is not to scale. The term 'homunculus' (mini human) in the quote above was popularised by the Montreal-based neurosurgeon Wilder Penfield. In the 1940s and 1950s he carried out electrical stimulation experiments on the somatosensory cortex of people who were awake, before they underwent surgery for epilepsy. He demonstrated convincingly how and where bodily sensations map on to the brain. As well as the right side of the body being mapped on to the left side of the brain, the scale is distorted. There are so many nerve endings coming from the tip of the forefinger, especially on the right if you are right-handed, that these require more brain space. The same applies to the tongue, lips and external genitalia, although their representation is still split in half along the vertical. The back and legs, in contrast, barely merit space at all. But there is also a motor homunculus controlling movement, not in the parietal lobe but further forward in the motor part of the frontal lobe. Here the fingers (and thumb) loom large and the legs and arms get at least some of the limelight commensurate with their action roles.[11]

So the body's images in the brain are drawn from the body in reality but differ from it. And this is only the start. As we move from the body as directly controlled and perceived, to the body as more vaguely 'felt' and into the body as imagined, we move from the tangibility of the physical world through psychology into the changeable and sometimes harsh realities of the social world. Each map or image becomes increasingly less literal as it passes from the somatosensory cortex to areas of the brain like the temporal and frontal lobes, where information to and from the body is not simply relayed but also manipulated and abstracted.

While neurological disorders of body schema tend to be lateralised and asymmetrical, the kind of disorders directed towards the neuropsychiatrist or psychiatrist and those which draw people to cosmetic surgeons are, in contrast, strikingly symmetrical focusing on the midline of the body: the nose, breasts, tummy, penis or overall size.

***

The next two sessions carried on along similar lines. Caitlín attended on time despite avoiding public transport, often wearing the same clothes. I tried to focus on her weight and physical health. She couldn't say what her weight was (she never weighed herself) but I guessed it was between six and seven stones (about eighty-five to a hundred pounds). She didn't care what she looked like and avoided spending time in front of the mirror. She let slip that she even avoided bathing until it was absolutely necessary. But she wasn't losing weight, at least not obviously. She wasn't menstruating; her weight was still below a critical level that evolution had decided would permit safe reproduction and trigger another homeostatic cascade starting from the hypothalamus, to switch on the ovaries. Her response was, "What do I need periods for, anyway?"

Her life followed a rigid routine of work and sleep, and she claimed to only need two meals a day. I was far from understanding what kept Caitlín going. My mind was crowded with uninvited food metaphors. Our sessions were bland. She would occasionally throw me scraps, but where was the beef? After our last meeting, I experienced a real – not at all metaphorical – craving for a bacon sandwich and just had to go to the local greasy spoon. Had talking about food piqued my appetite, or was it some sort of unconscious projection? Caitlín seemed immune from the normal feelings of hunger but had somehow transferred them to me. I needed to get to know her better so that she was not a mere conveyor of raw feelings but a real, three-dimensional person. I needed to put flesh on the bones.

Before my next appointment with Caitlín, I dug out some
old letters and notes from the file. She had had some counselling in her mid-twenties and subsequently, and sporadically,
more in-depth psychotherapy. Obviously, that was something
to explore.

The next session began much like the others, except she was
carrying a satchel stuffed with papers – part of her research.
She was wearing the usual drab, shapeless clothes and was still
gaunt. I took up her personal history where we had left off. She
had thrown herself into university and was drawn to modern
history, particularly the Second World War. This was still her
area of interest. She got a good degree, stayed on as a research
assistant and then embarked on a PhD. It had taken ages to
complete, but she had finally done so and was now a lecturer.
She was working on a book. Her subject was how institutions
in Europe, such as the Church and the Red Cross, reacted to
the rise of fascism.

I confessed my ignorance and asked her to say a little about
it. She perked up. Evidently she was more comfortable talking
about a topic where *she* was 'the expert' and she wasn't focusing
on her inner feelings. Academics in her field, she explained,
were often drawn to the obscure recesses of history and geogra-
phy, to incidents that might illuminate the bigger picture. She
had started out exploring the Balkans and had travelled there
extensively for her PhD.

She explained how various Croatian groups sided with the
Nazis and about atrocities visited upon the Serbs and Roma.
Had I heard of the Ustashe? I hadn't, and she shook her head
in disappointment. This was a violent nationalist movement

which grew in the interwar years, finally coming to power under the auspices of Nazi Germany but which proved too bloodthirsty and fanatical even for them. Their militias were notorious for the torture and grotesque mutilation of their victims. She described how they had garnered support from the Roman Catholic Church for their anti-Orthodox stance, which to this day had not been fully acknowledged – something that she felt personally ashamed of, having been brought up as Catholic.

It was a fascinating if disturbing history lesson. Was she trying to convey something to me symbolically via these accounts? There were several possibilities. What I took from them was that Caitlín had a fierce intelligence and an acute sensitivity to injustice and hypocrisy. I shouldn't underestimate her. The time passed, our half an hour was up. I remembered our ostensible purpose. How was her eating? Had she put on any weight? She wasn't sure about the texture of cream cheese – she had been moving towards veganism, she said – but she would persist. She'd put on a couple of pounds. It was neither here nor there. I said well done and recommended stretching the rules about two meals a day; for instance, having some nuts in between – something healthy and vegan too! She said she would try it, gathered up her stuff and left.

Our next appointment was a month later and I set aside an hour. I wasn't sure if it was my imagination, but she looked ever so slightly better, still very thin but with a bit more colour in her cheeks. She said she was tired, but her work was going well. She was finding out more about the Red Cross. Did I know that before the war, the Nazis took over the

German Red Cross and made it another part of their machine? The International Red Cross Committee, in the meantime, had to try to work around them and somehow support prisoners of war and concentration camp inmates with their famous 'food parcels'. I put to her that while I was genuinely interested in her work and we could easily fill the time with her giving me seminars, that might be a distraction. She stopped talking and looked deflated. Then she sat up, folded her arms and addressed me as if I was one of her less able students.

"So, what do you think we should be talking about?"

"Well, I was meaning to ask you...there was a mention in your records about having counselling."

"Oh, that. I saw someone regularly for a bit. She was a psychotherapist, actually really helpful. It seems like a long time ago. Do we have to go into it again?"

"No, we don't have to, but I was wondering what prompted it."

"Oh, you know...I didn't like myself and I didn't like the world." She paused a long time. "It was when I was travelling round the former Yugoslavia. I met an English guy. He'd dropped out of uni and was bumming around Europe. I liked him. I thought we were friends. One evening he got drunk and forced... He sexually assaulted me. It wasn't technically rape, so I was told. It was still...disgusting. The betrayal of trust...put me off sex...and men...and people, if I'm honest."

Caitlín was calm, almost matter-of-fact.

"Sounds awful. Did you report it or seek help at the time?"

"No; no point. Anyway, I'm over it."

A revelation like this is always hard to digest. Despite her attempt to downplay the event, it seemed self-evidently relevant and important. However, I felt I had to resist the temptation to believe that it somehow solved everything, that it was the one answer, the hidden mystery, that no further explanation was required. It was bound to be more complicated than that. Hesitantly, I picked up the thread.

"Are you really over it?"

"Yes," she said emphatically. "For a time I was self-harming; I cut myself." She pointed to her chest. "It was really bad. But now I realise it was not my fault. I do not have to feel guilty. And I haven't given up on men; well, not completely... But it did put my life in perspective. What happened to me is nothing compared with what others, especially women, endured during the war. Things people take for granted...food, shelter, love... Well, you can't, you shouldn't."

I carefully formulated a response. "So, if you deny yourself those things, then no one else can deny you them."

"No, you're not getting it. I'm not like other people. I really don't need them."

Could that be true? Caitlín was consistent if nothing else. She didn't need to enjoy food and she didn't expect to be happy, and this gave her a feeling of being different from other people, possibly even superior.

We had run out of time again. Before we finished, I asked her about her eating. The nuts were OK, she said.

"So how about dipping the apple in a bit of honey?"
"Ugh!" She grimaced. "I'll have a go."

*****

The emotion of disgust is based on avoidance of contamination.[12] The word is related to that for taste in French (*dégoût*) and Latin (*gustare*), and the meaning is similar to 'distaste' in English. The quintessential disgusting experience is eating human or animal waste. Just the mention of it will produce a 'yuk' response with the characteristic facial expression of shutting the mouth firmly, expelling its contents by sticking out the tongue and bottom lip and closing the nostrils to smells, or in the extreme, gagging. Looking at facial expressions of disgust activates the brain areas involved in taste. But what is so interesting about disgust is how it has accrued other, more extensive triggers. Most simply, any bodily fluid or substance can elicit a response of disgust. It doesn't have to be taken in the mouth; any contact may do it. Furthermore, the act of taking into the body extends to sexual behaviour, which can also elicit a strong response, positive and erotic or negative and repellent. In fact, disgust is perhaps unique in generating so many taboos and rituals which pervade culture (e.g. dietary laws in religion, cleaning rituals, rules about sex and menstruation, and so forth). What started as a mechanism to limit contagion has evolved to define the boundaries between us – our kith and kin and loved ones, whose waste and secretions we are inclined to tolerate, and even our wider social group, whose ideas and values (if not bodily fluids) we are happy to share. We commonly express moral outrage by saying we are disgusted. Psychological experiments have shown that people will recoil if asked to taste some fruit juice served up in a bed pan, albeit brand new and unused, and show a similar automatic aversive physical response to, say, an item of Nazi uniform.[13]

Some psychiatric syndromes can be viewed as disgust based: fears of contamination are at the core of obsessive–compulsive disorder, leading to compulsive washing and avoidance of 'dirt'. Eating disorders have this quality too.[14] While avoiding calories may be the central motive, many people would retch at the thought of a rare-cooked steak dripping in blood and fat. Indeed, many of us are increasingly troubled by our diets, both out of a need to avoid putting on weight and out of concern for the environment. It's increasingly unclear where a healthy concern tips into an unhealthy fixation with what we are putting in our mouths: its provenance, its purity, its health-giving properties, its potential as an allergen. Some authorities have coined the term orthorexia ('correct' eating) to describe this new phenomenon.[15]

***

The next couple of sessions continued as before. In the time we had, Caitlín updated me on her research and the book; we usually finished with a review of what she was consuming day to day. She was definitely putting on weight now and noted that, paradoxically, the more she did so the less she was preoccupied with eating the correct things. She had started wearing clothes in colours other than black and khaki, and instead of walking the three miles to the clinic, she had started taking the bus. Her manner remained detached and, emotionally, she remained distant. Could we do better than putting it all down to an 'atypical eating disorder'? Clearly when I first saw her, she was eating a highly restricted diet which was having adverse physiological effects. Her clothes and bearing hinted at some body-image problems, in that she had projected herself as shapeless and uncomfortable in her own skin. Now she seemed more at ease in her body. As for depression, she did have anhedonia, but it was more than that. She saw no reason to take pleasure in food because her ultimate aim was not the pursuit of happiness. She felt burdened by the horrors that she had uncovered through researching wartime Europe and felt she had to honour the victims in some way. I began to see her not so much as a patient suffering from an eating disorder but as a true ascetic, carrying the sins of humanity, seeking to live a good and simple life and asking nothing in return. I had to respect her for that.

Some scholars propose that the earliest manifestations of anorexia nervosa are seen clearly in the Middle Ages in the lives of the saints, in women whose self-denial and even self-flagellation was termed 'holy anorexia'.[16] But there was nothing histrionic about Caitlín's self-denial. It was a moral choice arising out of her analysis of recent history and contemporary life: an amoral present and immoral past.

Psychiatrists have to guard against making moral judgements, but that is a nearly impossible task. The overweight and obese are one of the most reviled groups on earth, even though they are quickly becoming the majority. Some people with anorexia nervosa, if they are being honest, will admit to really despising fat people and attributing to them all the worst characteristics (i.e. lazy, smelly, feckless, slothful and greedy). It would be quite reprehensible were it not for the fact that they reserve the worst opprobrium for themselves. And just as the deployment of size-zero fashion models has drawn criticism for the way it distorts young people's sense of what they should look like, under the radar, the hedonic-homeostatic battle in eating is exploited by advertising for foodstuffs with their use of the language of temptation, sinfulness and 'naughty but nice' strap lines.[17]

I was still searching for the bigger picture. Was Caitlín's disorder really a lifestyle choice, or was she identifying with the female victims of the Ustashe? What about her sexual assault? While 'technically not rape', what kind of intrusion was she forced to endure? And let's not forget her family life: losing her father at a critical time and the knock-on effects on her mother, whom she may feel she had abandoned. In addition, there were consistent themes running through her research, something about institutions that should be beyond reproach, nurturing and protective: the sanctuary of the Church and the Red Cross, each a rare source of goodness amidst the horrors of war – what a psychoanalyst might call the ultimate 'good breast' – both turning out to be horribly tainted. Was it possible to pull it all together?

I looked forward to speaking to her and learning from her, but despite that, I also thought it might be time to discharge her from the clinic. She agreed. (She had been thinking about that herself.)

"So what do we conclude?" she said in lecturer mode.

I began by saying I thought that due to her upbringing and some difficult experiences, she didn't believe she deserved to experience pleasure through the ways that others do quite naturally, such as enjoying food, because it always went wrong. I put forward my psychodynamic interpretation of her thesis and historical research and ended by saying it was now up to her whether she was going to be a prisoner of history or whether she was going to write her own.

After a pause, she said she thought that was 'interesting' and that 'I may have a point'. In fact, she had some news. She was in the early phases of her first 'proper' relationship. He was much older, divorced – and her head of department. It would probably be frowned on by the university.

"Another example of something good being tainted, as you would say. Anyway, thanks for your help."

And with that, she said goodbye.

I felt strangely empty. One doesn't honestly expect an interpretation, regardless of how well honed, to come as a true revelation: *yes, of course! All is clear. Why didn't I see that before?* Rather, I believe the best interpretations produce a perturbation in thinking. It's not about proving something right, but instead that it brings about a new way of seeing the problem, usually because it's *almost* right. But to be greeted with mild indifference…

The patient had got better, which was fine, but I had ventured out of my depth. I should not have pretended I was a psycho-analyst. I'm a neuropsychiatrist. Or a dietician, at a push.

***

About a year later, Caitlín phoned out of the blue, asking if she could see me. Of course I agreed, fearing the worst. She bounded in, looking untidy but radiant. She said, "I want you to meet Francis, my partner." Francis shyly stepped forward. He was balding and slightly overweight, wearing a crumpled suit. He exuded calm and generosity. He shook my hand saying, "I've heard a lot about you." How embarrassing.

"Oh yes," Caitlín continued as she wheeled in a buggy, "and this is Matthew, our new baby."

6

Silent Music

It was an eerie place. A small, self-contained ward with half a dozen beds, bleached by artificial light. Green LED screens displayed oscillating waveforms, emitting rhythmical beeps. Staff in starched uniforms with clipboards, making notes, speaking softly. Cuddly toys, enlarged colour photographs stuck on the walls: young people gurning for selfies; bungee jumps; celebration cakes with twenty-one candles.

This was a unit for people in a persistent vegetative state (PVS) or minimally conscious state (MCS). All had suffered 'catastrophic brain damage'. (For once, the technical term is not a euphemism but tells it like it is.) For the younger people the catastrophe is mostly a traumatic one, a road-traffic accident, sometimes described in medical-note shorthand as 'lorry vs man' or 'car vs bike'. Occasionally it's encephalitis, a viral infection of the brain. Across the age range, brain haemorrhage or tumours – and overzealous neurosurgery – can do it. Another major cause is anoxia (lack of oxygen) to the brain following cardiac arrest, strangulation (perhaps following a suicide attempt by hanging), drowning or a major metabolic upset such as prolonged hypoglycaemia (low blood sugar due to a diabetic person getting way too much insulin). There are also many individually rare causes, such as inherited disorders affecting the fundamental biochemical processes or those leading to degeneration of the brain tissue, which add up in aggregate.

***

I was advising on a forty-two-year-old patient, Malik, with schizophrenia. He had recently fallen or jumped from a three-storey building and sustained a severe head injury. He was emerging slowly from a coma and was now shouting out occasionally and pulling at his feeding tube, seemingly distressed. He had been on maintenance antipsychotic medication, but the team looking after him wasn't sure if he should go back on it. It was the sort of fair question often asked of the neuropsychiatrist but for which there is almost no reliable guidance available from clinical trials. Was he really 'distressed' or was his body merely reacting in a reflexive way to the intrusive life support? Were his schizophrenia – or his suicidal impulses, if he had them – beginning to reassert themselves now that he was recovering consciousness? It was impossible to tell. The patient's elderly mother was hovering by the door and caught my eye.

"Is he going to all right, doctor?"

She was well spoken with just a hint of a South Asian accent. She came across as educated; polite but direct. I explained that I wasn't part of his clinical team so wasn't the best person to speak to, realising that this sounded evasive.

"You're the neuropsychiatrist, aren't you?"

"Yes, but—"

"You know Malik has had mental health problems for years, since he was a young man… He's been on tablets and injections for ages."

"Yes, right, and I think he probably should go back on them…although it's hard to say if they will help, and they might even interfere with him coming round. You see, we really don't know what the best thing to do is for people in your son's situation—"

"I understand that, it's just that I was wondering, is there any chance that…you'll probably say I'm stupid, but is there any chance that he might, you know…be better now? They used to do brain operations for schizophrenia, lobotomies, so maybe this will have damaged the bad bits, the mad bits, and now he might be better off. It's like when they tell you to switch the computer off and on again. Sometimes that does the trick!"

I hadn't seen that coming. Such was this poor mother's desperation that maybe, just maybe, she allowed herself to believe, a catastrophic brain injury could have a plus side.

As I continued towards the exit I was distracted again. There was a young woman in her late teens, or perhaps early twenties, in the last bed, lying flat on her back, arms outstretched over the covers, her eyelids flickering. A bag of white liquid hung on a stand, connected via a thin tube to her belly. A junior doctor was by her side, leaning over her.

"Emma, Emma, are you OK?"

No response. The flickering paused for a few seconds and then resumed.

"Emma…anybody home?"

Nothing. Then the doctor gently, with his forefinger and thumb, pulled the patient's eyelids towards the forehead effectively forcing the eyes open. The patient's eyeballs then rolled upwards exposing the white sclerae. This is called Bell's phenomenon and is a normal reflex response that happens when a person closes their eyes. Here, it shows that the person is actively resisting having their eyes opened for them and strongly suggests that they are awake and alert, despite appearances. The doctor shrugged, stroked Emma's eyes closed again and turned to walk away. I beckoned him over.

"What's the matter with *her*?" I whispered.

The doctor shook his head. "Nobody knows."

Later I called the consultant. We discussed Malik and his medication and agreed a plan. But before I put the phone down, I couldn't resist asking about Emma. The consultant was an expert in rehabilitation medicine, but she was neither a neurologist nor a psychiatrist, and she admitted being baffled by Emma's presentation.

"I was dying to get you or one of your colleagues to see her," she said, "but Emma's in the middle of a court case. Her dad doesn't want her to have any more investigations. He thinks they will make her worse, but the local authority disagrees, so it will be up to a judge to decide."

***

Severe damage or disruption to the brain, short of death, may result in coma. This is defined as an unarousable state of unresponsiveness. Despite vigorous efforts on the part of their attendants, the victim does not open their eyes and shows 'no evidence of awareness of the self or environment'.[1] There is a grizzly hierarchy of terms that eventually lead from coma to full conscious awareness. The lowest rung on the ladder is the vegetative state, where so-called vegetative functions – circulation, breathing, digestion – carry on as normal, as it were, regardless. In this state the person does open their eyes and, at times, looks as if they are undergoing a sleep–wake cycle of sorts. Nevertheless, some might question how much of the person is actually there. They show no reproducible, purposeful behaviour. They don't respond to sensory stimulation such as loud noises, flashing lights, exhortations, pinching and poking (apart from reflex spasms). There is no evidence of language comprehension nor expression, and again, that deathly phrase: no evidence of awareness of the self or environment. In the UK, this starts to be called persistent if it continues for more than a month and permanent for more than six months (or a year following traumatic brain injury). Emerging from this state as some do leads to the next rung, minimally conscious state, defined as some purposeful behaviour – even if rare and inconsistent. That might mean a response to sensory stimulation, a show of awareness, or some rudimentary two-way communication. The rung after that is where there is more consistent, but still severely limited, behaviour such as being able to grab an object when offered, carry out a simple command, or to show recognition, pleasure or pain to a familiar face or sound, and perhaps utter a few words or phrases. This is the realm of severe disability. These diagnoses should only be made after thorough and repeated assessments over days and weeks supplemented by knowledge of what happened to lead to the situation in the first place.

Although there are no simple tests to establish PVS or MCS, because they need to explore all sensory modalities and be repeated, usually these individuals will have been extensively analysed, X-rayed and scanned, often in the course of heroic attempts to resuscitate them.[2]

Such scans and investigations show extensive disruption of the brain. In the final reckoning, the post-mortem examination, sometimes coming years after the terrible event, shows this in close-up. In addition to whatever blows, bleeds or blockages have been meted out to the brain, a common feature following trauma is 'diffuse axonal injury', the widespread shearing of nerve fibres throughout the white matter. Almost invariable is damage to the thalamus, the critical relay station deep in the centre of the brain. The lack or virtual lack of consciousness may be attributed to that. Going lower down into the brain stem, which is responsible for those basic 'mechanical' vegetative functions, there will be fewer signs of damage (otherwise, the individual could not have survived).[3]

A cruel mimic of PVS and MCS is the 'locked-in syndrome'. In this, the person cannot speak or move at all, save for being able to blink, open their eyes and, classically, move them up and down at will. Inside this prison they are fully conscious and aware and can use their eye movements to communicate, albeit arduously, with the outside world. Such communication has resulted in a number of astounding autobiographical accounts, perhaps most famously *The Diving Bell and the Butterfly* by French former journalist Jean-Dominique Bauby.[4] The syndrome is caused by damage to the ventral pons, the front of the upper part of the brain stem, where the trunk of nerve fibres carrying instructions from the higher parts of the brain down to the rest of the body have been severed, usually by a very precise blood clot or haemorrhage. The fibres to the muscles which move the eyes up and down have left the main trunk just above that point and so are spared, but everything below is disconnected. Information coming into the brain from the rest of the body and the special senses (sight, sound, smell and taste) takes a different route so is also unaffected.

The thought of misdiagnosing locked-in syndrome for PVS is horrifying and that of misdiagnosing MCS for PVS, hardly less so. And yet the estimated rate of misdiagnosis for PVS is thought to be as high as 40%.[5] Often this is because major sensory deficits, such as blindness, complicate the assessment or because demonstrations of awareness are fleeting and almost imperceptible. Sadly, however, the opposite is also true, with deep understanding sometimes being attributed to random groans and grimaces. Who could blame loved ones, carers and sometimes highly trained staff for inferring conscious intention on the flimsiest pretext? Adrian Owen, a neuropsychologist working in Canada, and colleagues have produced startling research using functional MRI scans which show the brain in action by picking up tiny changes in blood flow to those parts of the brain engaged in a particular task.

They studied a twenty-three-year-old woman who was thought to be in a vegetative state following a car accident.

Five months into this state, the researchers were able to detect brain activity in the supplementary motor area (a fron tal brain region where motor plans are formed) whenever she was asked to imagine playing tennis, as well as activity in a very different region, the parahippocampal gyrus (the region believed to create and store maps of familiar environments), whenever she was imagining walking around her home.[6] This provided an elaborate basis for answering yes and no to a series of questions, proving that she had sufficient conscious awareness to communicate meaningfully. We instinctively use conversation and the ebb and flow of question and answer to infer what a person thinks and believes. That this requires conscious awareness is something we take for granted but has been much debated by philosophers and computer scientists specialising in artificial intelligence, as in the famous Turing Test.[7] Using the MRI scanner to produce pictures of the working brain is cumbersome and requires highly complex hardware and software. Work to translate these findings into a simple clinical test is ongoing.

***

Of course, Emma did not reach this point all of a sudden. There was a long descent. She was an only child, born after her mother, Miranda, had suffered several miscarriages, so Emma was especially cherished. She was a frail and premature baby who spent her first few weeks in a special-care baby unit, circumstances that again may have set in train a pattern of parent–child interaction, which heightened their view of her as vulnerable and needing extra protection. Nevertheless, she developed normally and attended ordinary school. She was generally a little above average academically and had a tight circle of friends but was clumsy and very bad at games. As she progressed through school, her parents often found themselves fighting battles with the authorities. The first one was to have her assessed for 'apraxia', which replaced clumsiness as a descriptor and entitled her to remedial help and extra time at exams because of her poor handwriting.

The transition from junior to high school was especially challenging for Emma. 'Big school' was an intimidating environment and Emma often ended up in the sick bay with the school nurse because of headaches, feeling sick and, later, fatigue. Things were not good at home either. Her mum, an artist, had decided to leave the home to join an ashram. Both parents had come to the view that they were incompatible. Emma's dad, Charles, was a senior civil servant working in government and had expected his wife to play a more conventional role as homemaker but instead found himself being the person who did the school run, attended the parents' evenings and helped with the homework. Miranda found him to be increasingly rigid and believed that children were put under too much pressure at school and that this dulled their creativity. On top of that, Charles had had serious health problems, being diagnosed with an aggressive form of lymphoma. He had undergone surgery and chemotherapy but was told that his prognosis was not good since the cancer had already spread to his bone marrow and possibly his lungs. He looked into the options and found that further chemotherapy at his stage had a low chance of success and so declined further treatment, much to the annoyance and dismay of his oncologist. Nearly ten years on, he was still alive and well. He had changed his diet and against his usually hyper-rational instincts had become interested in herbal remedies. He wasn't going to claim that this had brought about a miracle cure, but it did undermine his faith in medical authority and orthodox treatments. It seemed that the doctors didn't know everything after all.

All the while, Emma's health problems got worse. Sometimes she outright refused to go to school, saying she felt she was about to faint and was exhausted. She was already being excused from physical education and Charles wondered whether there was a deeper problem at school, bullying perhaps, but found no evidence of this. Things got worse. He took her a number of times to the general practitioner (GP), who couldn't find anything wrong. The GP was someone the family had known since Emma was born. She was dedicated and they trusted her. She even gave Emma some one-to-one meetings and made sure there was nothing untoward going on at home. She said Emma was growing and developing normally. She did some blood tests including one for glandular fever. The latter came back positive, but that just meant that she had at some point contracted the virus (along with 90% of her peers). The GP thought she would grow out of it but was sympathetic to Emma's situation. It wasn't easy being a young girl going through puberty without your mother and no doubt worrying whether your father was going to stick around.

Charles didn't want to accept such explanations – it was clearly a physical problem – and he couldn't help feeling he was being blamed for Emma's condition. He seemed to spend as much time with the school nurse as with Emma's teachers. The nurse said that a pattern was emerging: if they did manage to get Emma to school, she was fine until early afternoon when she just seemed to fade and often had to be sent home. The nurse wondered about chronic fatigue syndrome (CFS) or myalgic encephalomyelitis (ME). Charles looked it up on the internet. He was surprised, shocked even, by the amount of stuff out there. Some of it was quite wacky – fad diets, allergies, 'experts' in America offering radical cures – but much of it rang true. The advice from the self-help groups to sufferers was clear: don't try to force yourself to carry on, you will just make it worse. You need to pace yourself. For children, if home schooling is an option, take it. Most doctors don't 'know best'; they are largely ignorant, or they think it's all in the mind, not a real illness; that it's just 'psychiatric'. Worryingly, there were numerous blogs posted from people who had become severely disabled, bedridden and tube fed.

Charles decided to get involved. He was well connected: he knew a number of Members of Parliament; he knew how bureaucracies worked. He started campaigning for better support and more flexibility from the school, for more holistic treatments on the NHS, for a more sympathetic benefits system. He could see that Emma was deteriorating and it seemed to be true: the more the school insisted on her

participating with the other healthy kids, the more she deteriorated. She started to withdraw, spending more time in her
bedroom, often with the curtains drawn and with headphones
on to block out noise, only getting up to go to the toilet.
Anything more and she felt dizzy and drained of energy. He
tried to talk to her. She didn't seem depressed; she wanted to
be 'normal', but she had ME. When the GP suggested a psychiatric referral to Emma, she refused; instead, Charles got her
admitted to a private hospital that specialised in CFS. It was
going to use up the family savings but would surely be worth it.
They took her seriously and did more blood tests, which
pointed to an immune problem, but it wasn't clear-cut and
didn't point to any treatment. They allowed Emma to set her
own goals. They let her use a wheelchair if it meant she could
attend the therapy sessions, and they did not force her to join
in if she didn't feel up to it.

Twelve months passed. Emma would have to forgo her A
levels. She barely got out of bed and spoke only a few words
before feeling too tired and falling asleep. Charles had run out
of money. The unit was giving mixed messages. Maybe Emma
was going to be one of the 25% who didn't get better; or maybe
she didn't *want* to get better. Could it be psychiatric after all?
Charles was outraged but bottled it up. He decided to take her
home. He would fight to get the help he needed: regular carers
and domiciliary nurses, a special bed and hoists. He would
work part-time and look after Emma himself, if necessary. By
this time, the battle lines were already being drawn. The GP
did not agree with the approach and proposed that the dizzi-
ness was the consequence, rather than the cause, of her

spending so much time in bed. The doctor pointed to Emma's lack of muscle mass: no wonder she felt weak. She needed to gradually build that up again and to be reassured that, in the long run, she would recover, even though it felt like activity was making her more tired in the short term. The doctor refused to sanction domiciliary nursing and instead wanted to give her a trial of antidepressants. The school was worried about all the education she had missed. The local authority was alerted. There were mutterings about 'safeguarding'. Wasn't it a bit weird for a father and daughter to be so close?

Charles had the downstairs living room turned into a bedroom for Emma with all the necessary adaptations for a disabled person. He paid for private carers. Some of Emma's friends would visit, but they felt awkward telling their stories of nights out, boyfriends and plans to go to university, and soon they stopped coming. Often she would spend the evening gently sobbing into her pillow. The local patient support group were the only outsiders on whom Charles could rely. They were always there for him.

Weeks later, in the middle of the night, Charles woke up to find Emma, who had somehow fallen out of bed, on the floor. She seemed to be having some kind of fit. He called the ambulance and they took her to A&E.

After an upsetting night in the hospital emergency department, they diagnosed 'non-epileptic attacks'. She was admitted and given a full medical examination – pulse, blood pressure, chest, heart and abdomen – all normal. The neurological examination, such as it was with an uncooperative patient, was normal. Reflexes were also normal. A routine electroencephalogram (EEG) and computed tomography brain scan were done the next day and were both normal. So was the electrocardiogram. Blood tests were repeated and they too came back normal, except for signs of dehydration. However, Emma looked far from normal. She remained unresponsive and incontinent. Lying flat in bed, she was now floppy as a rag doll. Her eyes were closed, the lids occasionally flickering, and she did not speak, even with her father. She was getting liquids and nutrition via a tube going into her stomach through her nose. The nursing staff tried everything they could think of to encourage her to sit up and communicate, but to no avail.

Two weeks went by. The psychiatric team were called in. They said that given the history and deterioration, Emma should be admitted to a psychiatric unit for adolescents. Charles was not entirely happy with this direction. He would have preferred the medical team to acknowledge that Emma had CFS and that she needed time to recover.

Nonetheless, after a few days, the child and adolescent psychiatrist visited. He spent time with Charles and Emma on their own and spoke to the GP and nursing staff. He suggested further esoteric tests for rare metabolic abnormalities and toxins (tests which came back clear). He wrote in his notes that he had never seen a case quite like this before but that it reminded him of pervasive refusal syndrome (PRS).[8]

The syndrome, described as recently as 1991 by British child psychiatrist Bryan Lask,[9] begins in a similar way to Emma's condition but reaches a point where the child overtly refuses to move or talk (although they may choose to talk to certain people, usually when out of sight of family or carers). The child refuses to eat regularly and, sometimes, to use the toilet. Unlike Emma's case, the refusal is more active and occasionally angry, even aggressive. They will turn away if approached, rolling over in bed or huddling up in a ball. If an attempt is made to get them up or turn them in one direction, they will pull themselves in the opposite direction and may shout or whine. The syndrome affects girls more than boys. The children are described as coming from middle-class backgrounds, being conscientious or even perfectionistic, and being emotionally 'enmeshed' with one or both parents. PRS may be triggered by stress or physical illness. Treatment often entails hospitalisation, especially if the patient is losing weight but also to create some distance between child and parent. A gradual process of gentle encouragement and exploration of the child's fears and concerns, plus physical rehabilitation, seems to be effective but may take many months. PRS is controversial insofar as it is a distinct syndrome rather than a manifestation of, say, severe depression, social anxiety, anorexia nervosa or psychosis, or an understandable reaction to social circumstances such as physical or sexual abuse.

Unfortunately for Emma, she was nearly eighteen years old at this point and the adolescent unit was reluctant to take someone of that age who was no longer attending school. The advice was that she should be referred for treatment on an adult psychiatry ward. Charles was having none of it. The child psychiatrist had to concede that an acute general psychiatric ward was not the place for someone with Emma's condition. Meanwhile the medical ward managers asserted that she was 'blocking a bed'. Charles decided to put his foot down. The stress of this episode and lack of any worthwhile treatment had been horrendous for Emma and had evidently worsened her condition. She was not having any more tests. She was not going to waste time with any more psychiatrists. He was taking her home.

The hospital staff, mental health team, safeguarding team, social workers and legal advisers all sprang into action. She couldn't go home in this condition with a nasogastric tube, dependent for all her care needs, with no management plan. It was an impasse. Lawyers were instructed and argued over the rights of the child, her capacity to make a decision, her best interests, the rights of the father, the Mental Health Act and Mental Capacity Act, her right to refuse treatment and her right to receive treatment. After weeks of wrangling, a bed on a 'High Dependency Brain Injury Unit' was found as an interim measure until a longer-term solution could be found – which is where I came in.

***

Several months passed before a High Court judge ruled that Emma be admitted to a neurological hospital for a limited time for investigations to determine the nature of her condition and to recommend treatment. It took three weeks. Every conceivable bodily fluid, including blood, urine and cerebrospinal fluid, was tested to rule out metabolic problems, infection or immune disturbance. A muscle biopsy was normal. An MRI scan showed the brain and spinal cord to be of normal appearance.

Electroencephalography was performed. This is a measure of faint electrical activity generated in the brain. Dozens of tiny wires are stuck onto the scalp which detect voltages, which are combined to create a map or 'montage' of brain activity. The EEG is the definitive means of detecting an epileptic seizure, which produces a burst of asynchronous spikes on the EEG record. It is also very useful in displaying a signature of conscious and unconscious states. The resting EEG, a mass of indecipherable squiggles to the casual observer, can be decomposed electronically into recognisable wavebands with characteristic frequencies. The alpha band has a frequency of 8–13 Hz and is the rhythm of consciousness. It is best detected by leads attached to the back half of the scalp and is most clear when the person has their eyes closed and is relaxed. Theta has a frequency band from 4 up to 8 Hz, and the delta band has frequencies up to 4 Hz. These slower frequencies are undulating in the background but become prominent in cases of impaired consciousness. The EEG during sleep has its own set of stages and frequencies, but deep sleep is reflected in waves in the slower-frequency ranges without the tell-tale alpha band of consciousness. Frequencies above the alpha band are usually pathological and usually due to drug effects including intoxication. There is no characteristic EEG pattern that corresponds to PVS or MCS because there are often individual variations depending on which parts of the brain are damaged and to what extent, although it is usually highly deranged. What we do know is that the presence of a normal alpha rhythm is incompatible with coma or PVS.[10] The hospital carried out EEG monitoring over several days so as to capture the episodes of eye fluttering and other occasional movements that Emma displayed (because they might well have been epileptic seizures), as well as her sleep. The EEG showed a good alpha rhythm and, like every other test we had thrown at Emma, looked completely normal throughout. According to these results, her brain was physically healthy and conscious.

We had one other test up our sleeve. The principles behind the EEG can also be used to measure evoked or event-related potentials. These are waveforms which follow tens of milliseconds after a stimulus. The stimulus could be a flash of light, an auditory tone or any sensory event; or a more complex sequence of stimuli, such as a series of tones at one pitch interspersed with the occasional tone at another, all the way up to pictures of people and places, familiar or unfamiliar, written or spoken words or sentences. The stimuli are repeated several times so that the evoked waveform can be averaged out against the background activity. Consistent waveforms or potentials occurring up to around 150 milliseconds (msec) after the stimulus show early sensory perception and do not imply any conscious awareness, whereas those occurring beyond 250 msec (i.e. a quarter of a second) imply a degree of complex processing. So if we were to play a sequence of tones at the same pitch followed by one that was out of key, we would expect to see a characteristic positive waveform at around 300 msec after the surprise tone,[11] implying that we had foxed the subject's expectations; or if we were to read the subject a seemingly meaningful sentence that ended with an inappropriate word, we should see a negative electrical deviation at 400 msec or more from the moment that word begins, again implying deeper and perhaps more 'thoughtful' processing. There is no exact time point at which you could say a conscious mind emerges from the workings of the remarkable neural processor churning away outside of consciousness, but those later reactions would seem to depend on conscious awareness.[12]

Emma was subjected to bright flashing lights that evoke a response even when a person's eyes are closed. These responses proved to us that her brain was at least registering visual stimuli, and we found the same for equivalent tests in the auditory domain. A stream of spoken English words evoked a very different response to acoustically equivalent non-words. Experts from all the specialties came to see and examine her like visiting Magi and opined. Not one of the tests or one of the experts concluded that she had brain damage. It wasn't that she might have some form of damage or a disease the nature or cause of which was unknown; no, everything pointed towards a healthy body and a healthy nervous system. Surely, this had to be a psychiatric disorder. There is a false dichotomy between 'real' medical conditions and 'unreal' psychiatric ones, but it is a line of reasoning that frequently plays out. A psychiatrist, working with the neurology team, was also asked to give an opinion. After collating the now voluminous records and statements, they concluded that Emma was not suffering from an undiagnosed medical disease but instead had a psychiatric condition. It was possibly PRS (noting the caveats); possibly

an unusual form of depression known as 'depressive stupor';
possibly catatonia.[13] Given that she had shown no response to
high-intensity nursing care for the last three months, the only
intervention likely to be effective and which was indicated for
both depressive stupor and catatonia was electroconvulsive
therapy (ECT).

***

Most people get their picture of ECT from films such as *One
Flew Over the Cuckoo's Nest* (1975) with Jack Nicholson and
Changeling (2008) with Angelina Jolie. In the former film, the
ECT was given 'unmodified' (i.e. without a general anaesthetic), a practice abolished since the early 1950s and certainly
one much more frightening to watch. In *Changeling*, a true
story dating back to 1928, painstakingly recreated by director
Clint Eastwood, unmodified ECT is given to a mother (played
by Jolie) whose child has been abducted, a crime covered up
by the State. However, ECT was not invented until 1938. In
her book, *Cinema's Sinister Psychiatrists: From Caligari to
Hannibal*,[14] Dr Sharon Packer provides a possible non-polem-
ical explanation for filmmakers' apparent fascination with
ECT. The 'supposedly wild thrashing…[the] complicated
mechanical apparatus with flashing lights and mysterious
knobs… ECT scenes tell the audience that something special
is happening on screen'. Compare that with a nurse offering
the protagonist a couple of pills on a tray with a little cup of
water. It's not quite the same.

A study published in the *British Journal of Psychiatry* in 1980 found that 82% of 166 patients who had undergone ECT said it was the same or less upsetting than going to the dentist.[15] However, in 2003, Diana Rose, a service user researcher, published a meta-analysis in the *British Medical Journal*,[16] which analysed similar satisfaction surveys according to whether they were partly designed or initiated by service users (i.e. patients) versus doctors. She and her colleagues found that the former tended to show satisfaction levels below 50%. Either attitudes have changed over the intervening decades or it really matters who is asking the questions (probably both).

Out of all the controversial treatments in psychiatry, ECT is perhaps the most contested and one of the strangest.[17] It is, as mentioned, administered under a general anaesthetic (GA) with a muscle relaxant, usually in a suite within a psychiatric hospital designed for the purpose. As soon as the patient is anaesthetised, the 'paddles' are applied, either to each temple or both on the same side of the head, by the psychiatrist. A current is switched on for a few seconds until an epileptic seizure is induced. Muscle contraction is reduced to a minimum but not abolished, so the physical manifestation of the seizure is observed by the scrunching of the eyelids, tensing of the jaw and noticeable but not violent trembling of the limbs. This lasts about ten to forty seconds and then subsides. A minute or two later, the patient wakes up and may be a little dazed, but after a rest and a cup of tea, they will be ready to return to the ward or even to be taken home if they are an outpatient. ECT is usually prescribed, for reasons of convention, in courses of six and is usually administered two to three times per week for two to four weeks.

Because of the controversy that surrounds ECT as well as the need for a GA with its accompanying health risks and all the pala-ver, it tends to be reserved as a treatment of last resort where psychological therapies and medications have failed. Another consideration is where life is genuinely in danger – through dehy-dration or unrelenting suicidal urges. ECT is also indicated for the sort of diagnoses raised in Emma's case, sparingly in cases of schizophrenia (often where there is a large mood component and the medications are not working) or very, very rarely in mania.

But does it work? Attempts to put together all the results from all the old controlled clinical trials generally give a quali-fied 'yes' such that in the UK, the invariably cautious National Institute of Health and Care Excellence still recommends ECT in its guidelines for a few carefully chosen conditions and indi-cations.[18] However, there is a paucity of really good, large-scale studies with long-term follow-up (to see whether an initial benefit is sustained). There are many reasons for this, not least the formidable logistical difficulties in doing a randomised controlled trial where all the relevant patients have a severe and possibly life-threatening condition.[19]

Another big problem with ECT is the lack of a clear rationale for its use. Its original rationale was that epileptic seizures and psychosis were mutually incompatible, but that theory has been abandoned. When it comes to working out a biological mecha-nism for its therapeutic action, the problem is not that ECT doesn't produce measurable effects on neurotransmitter levels, brain hormones, neuronal growth factors, genes regulating brain metabolism and so forth; it's more that it does all of these things more or less indiscriminately. Whatever the current neurobiological theory is of, say, antidepressant treatment, you can bet that ECT will be found to do it too.

Finally, like any effective treatment, there is a balance to be struck between benefits and harms. ECT is clearly invasive, and inducing a fit, even under highly controlled conditions, would not normally be considered desirable. The main side effect is memory loss. While early studies find that, in the vast majority of cases this is temporary and inconsequential, work by Diana Rose and her colleagues suggests that the problem is much more common and sometimes persistent. One explanation for such contradictory views is that, when patients themselves are asked, they frequently note memory difficulties, but they do not – and cannot be expected to – distinguish whether such problems are due to the well-known impairment in memory that can accompany severe depression or due to the ECT. The best that can be said for ECT is that it produces an extra drain on a memory system that is already under pressure from the effects of depression, but that it might only be transient.

The results of all Emma's investigations and the conclusions reached by the neurologists and their colleagues were sent back to the court. After due deliberation, the judge ordered that the treatment plan proposed by the psychiatrist be taken forwards including a course of ECT, to be undertaken in a reputable psychiatric hospital as soon as one could be found that would take a person with Emma's considerable needs.

***

The irrepressibly cheerful Ghanaian healthcare assistant, Christiana, was a fixture on our ward. Her large billowing frame, along with a trolley teetering with jugs of water, flannels, detergents and towels, rolled along the hospital corridor from side room to side room. The bright yellow-and-orange floral scarf tied around her head clashed with the electric-blue disposable gloves she wore to do Emma's 'personal care' comprising a blanket bath, 'oral hygiene' and emptying her urinary-catheter bag. She and the nurse accompanying her would then do the usual measures of temperature, pulse and blood pressure. I came in towards the end one morning to observe. The routine took on the rhythm of the songs blaring out of the radio on the windowsill and had become a rather joyous dance. Emma lay there passively, eyes open, looking straight ahead. I noted that she seemed to cooperate with the washing and drying by rolling slightly to one side while a disposable sheet was squeezed under her body and then back again; imperceptibly raising each arm in anticipation of her armpits being wiped.

"C'mon sleeping beauty, you're going to be the belle of the ball," they joked as they combed her hair.

Christiana turned up the volume as the chords of a familiar favourite filled the room and sang along. "*Dancing queen, wash your face with some Windolene, oh yeah.*"

I could swear that Emma smiled, a broad grin playing across her face.

"Open wide, Lady Gaga," said Christiana.

Almost imperceptibly, Emma's lips parted, allowing Christiana to brush her teeth. How different this was from the controlled examination performed on Emma when she was first admitted! She would neither open nor close her mouth when asked, nor her eyes or fists. Sometimes her mouth would hang open. If a few drops of water were placed on her tongue, they would remain there a few seconds before trickling down the side of her mouth. And yet she did not dribble saliva (which continues to be produced throughout the day). This is unlike patients with catastrophic brain damage who risk choking, having lost the protective gag and swallowing reflexes and whose chins have to be constantly mopped.

***

Charles visited his daughter regularly. The interplay with the staff was edgy. He would question everything that was being done and they felt under surveillance. He was convinced that the efforts of the therapy team – occupational therapist, physiotherapist, ward psychologist – were misguided. They were following the approach recommended for kids with persistent refusal, which seemed to provide a reasonable template of gentle encouragement and praise without making demands, since that was thought to provoke resistance. Following his own sources, Charles, however, believed that even this might 'overload' Emma's body and would prolong her illness, which should be allowed to take whatever chronic course was its destiny. During his evening visits he would sit by her bed, stroking her hand. He would dim the light and switch off the TV. He didn't try to talk to her; in fact, he told her not to try to say anything.

The first meeting we arranged to discuss the treatment plan did not go well.

"Thank you for seeing me," said Charles, all formal courtesy.

He had come straight from work and was wearing a grey-pinstripe suit, white shirt and tie. I recapped where we were. The judge had persuaded Charles, on behalf of Emma, to put her fate in our hands. I explained that Emma could not be regarded as having the capacity to make decisions about her treatment, simply because she was, at the moment, unable to communicate. But rather than proceed with treatment in her best interests, as would be allowable under the Mental Capacity Act, my opinion was that this should be done under the Mental Health Act. I explained that ECT has special status within the Mental Health Act, requiring extra levels of independent scrutiny, which would help to protect her interests.

"How do you find her?" I enquired neutrally.

"As well as can be expected, under the circumstances."

He asked me what our working diagnosis was. I went through the list, the same one that had led the previous psychiatrist to recommend ECT. I explained that we had tried everything, including intramuscular benzodiazepine injections, the other treatment recommended for catatonia, as well as antidepressants and lots of physiotherapy, and had tried to get Emma to confide in us, all to no avail.

I said I was satisfied that we were not missing an underlying neurological condition. Emma was aware of what was going on around her and was able to act voluntarily but was doing her best to disguise this. Why? Only she knew.

"So you think she's putting it on?"

"No, that's not what I'm saying. I think she is suffering from a serious psychiatric disorder and that is why she is like she is, but I don't think she is physically incapable of speaking. And anyway, it's not helpful to consider things in such a dualistic way. The body and the mind are surely one and the same."

"And so you propose to shock her out of it." I let that go. "Have you, with all your experience and knowledge of philosophy, ever dealt with someone with Emma's condition?"

"Well, no one *quite* like her —"

"Yet you seem remarkably relaxed about using her as a human guinea pig!" His face was reddening. "How do you know it won't make her worse?"

"Worse? How could she possibly be worse? She was sharing a ward with people in a persistent vegetative state, people who had had massive brain injuries, and could have passed for one of them. *They* don't have any options open to them. And yes, I have seen people in a depressive stupor or catatonia 'waking up' after ECT and making a full recovery. Shouldn't we be giving Emma that chance?"

"You think I don't want the best for my daughter, after what we've been through? How dare you!"

He loosened his collar. I noticed the scar on his neck where a lymph node must have been removed when he had lymphoma. It was like a rebuke.

He collected himself. "You of all people should realise that stress is hugely damaging and can have physical effects on the body."

I nodded, thankful to have something upon which we could agree.

"Surely you know that viruses can remain dormant in the nervous system until reactivated by stress, such as the herpes simplex virus which causes cold sores and the zoster virus which causes chicken pox in children and can then come back if the immune system is compromised and cause shingles."

"Yes," I said, "but I'm not sure what this has to do with—"

"Emma had glandular fever, which is caused by the Epstein–Barr virus…which is also a herpes virus, is it not? So how do you know that her condition isn't due to that?"

So that was his theory.

"I see you've been on the internet. Let me reassure you that any kind of viral infection has been ruled out by extensive tests—"

"Or do you think your profession knows all there is to know about viral infections and the brain?"

"No, of course not, but—"

"And please don't patronise me."

"I can assure you that if it was a question of infection or immune disturbance, it would have been discovered. I mean, if it was something you could just Google, don't you think we would have found it? Not just me but several clever and thoughtful doctors have tried. But anyway, even if it was some sort of encephalitis that doctors don't understand, that somehow doesn't show up on any scan, or in the spinal tap, and doesn't affect the EEG, how does that explain the way she can sometimes show awareness, especially when she isn't being asked directly to show it? Surely you must have seen that for yourself. That does point to some other kind of disorder, one that is—"

"All in the mind? Let me tell you what I've seen for myself, the night Emma had that fit and ended up in A&E. They wheeled her immediately into the resuscitation area. I was terrified. I thought…well, I thought I was going to lose her. Emma was writhing from side to side. Every so often, the movements would get faster and she would tense up her arms with her fists banging on the mattress, left and right, up and down. The movements would subside again for a minute or two only to build up again. She was given oxygen to breathe. The casualty doctor approached her with a syringe drawn up ready. He put a Velcro tourniquet on her left arm, yanked it out straight and tried to find a vein. In the midst of her shaking she reached over with her right hand, ripped off the tourniquet and then thrashed more violently. You know what the doctor said then? 'Oh, so that's how we're going to play it, is it?' Like it was a game. He stepped back and gawped at her. Then he removed the oxygen mask. Her eyes were flickering and she was swinging her head from left to right. The doctor grabbed her chin to stop the movements. She opened her eyes and stared at him. Someone handed him a torch and he shone it in her eyes and put his face right up to hers. She swatted the torch away. So then he goes, 'Now come on, Emma. You're not having an epileptic seizure. I know you can hear me. I need you to control yourself…now!' The movements were abating; her legs were going in a sort of cycling motion but her arms were still. 'That's more like it,' he said smugly. A few minutes went by. I knew she still wasn't right; then, she let out a piercing scream and started fitting again, banging on the mattress. The doctor threw his hands up and barked, 'OK, call the psychs!', turned on his heels and stormed off. It went on like that all night."

"That does sound appalling," I said, noting how his description encapsulated all the cardinal features of non-epileptic attacks or 'dissociative seizures'.

"Nobody told me what was going on or explained anything. Some of the nurses were kind; they managed to get her to take a few sips of water and told her she was going to be OK. After that she lost the ability to swallow and to speak. We waited around for hours. I asked the charge nurse what was happening and he said that they were going to admit Emma overnight but that I would have to wait. 'We've got a lot of genuinely sick people in tonight,' he said. And when they did eventually get her up on the ward they made her some hot chocolate, but I told them she can't drink on her own and they said, if she's really thirsty, she'll drink. That's when I decided to take her home."

I really felt for Charles and was beginning to see things from his perspective.

"Look, I'm really sorry that you were treated like that," I said to him. "It's unacceptable. I'm afraid there is a stigma around mental illness that goes very deep and includes other doctors. We don't know why Emma is in this state – it's definitely real and definitely serious, life-threatening even – but maybe we should think of it as more of a software problem than a hardware problem."

He wasn't convinced.

"Next you'll be telling me that ECT is just like turning the computer off and on again."

He stood up, fixed his tie, we shook hands and he left.

***

It took a while to get all the necessary experts to see Emma and give a second opinion. Everyone was stumped; some asked for tests to be repeated 'just in case we'd missed something' and others were more confident in their judgements, but the unanimous view was that ECT was indicated, had a reasonable chance of success and could be given safely. At no point did Emma respond to questions or ask any of her own. One of the visiting experts put it to her bluntly: if she objected to having ECT, she should make it known now and that would probably be enough to halt the proceedings. We left a pen and paper by her bed in case she wanted to write something down when no one was around. I had several long 'conversations' with her where I would sit by her bedside and say what I thought: that whatever was going on in her mind, she must be truly desperate; that it might be hard to communicate with people now that she had remained mute for over a year; and that she might feel an added conflict about being true to herself, not letting her dad down and yet surely wanting to make decisions for herself. The day before her first session of ECT was planned, I said I guessed she might be terrified about it, but that I thought it could really help her find a way of getting out of this...trap. After a pause, her eyelids started fluttering and her body trembling. I said that I was interpreting that as her confirming how anxious she was and invited her to try to say something, anything, to make her real feelings known. The tremulousness increased. I put my hand on her forearm; it subsided. I said I bet she was wishing she had her mum there to talk to. Perhaps there was a tear in her eye, or was I imagining it? I sat there for nearly an hour, in case she spoke. She didn't.

***

I followed Emma into the ECT suite. She was wheeled in, strapped to a large chair tilted back to stop her sliding down. The procedure went smoothly. The anaesthetist confirmed that she had had 'a good seizure'. Some patients, especially with catatonia, respond after the first treatment. Sometimes that's all they need. In such circumstances, it is hard to know whether it is a physiological response to the GA, the ECT or a psychological response to the whole drama.

In the recovery area the ECT staff checked her vital signs and gently tried to rouse her. I warned them that she didn't normally say anything. She lay still as her breathing became less laboured. Her eyes flickered open but stared straight ahead.

"Emma, are you OK?" said the ECT nurse, waving her hand in front of her. She then made as if she was going to flick Emma in the eye.

Emma blinked but did not shift her gaze.

"That's it; done. You did great. Your father's outside; I'll tell him he can see you on the ward in a few minutes."

Emma showed no reaction; same the next time, and the next, and the next. The agreed protocol was for six ECTs and, if there was no benefit, to leave it at that.

The fifth treatment was carried out like the others. In major depression it is often after the first four or five that ECT starts to take effect. I hung around the suite and recovery area. Emma was waking up from the anaesthetic; she was coughing to expel some secretions from her lungs. The ECT nurse raised the top section of the recovery trolley so that she would be propped up in the sitting position. Emma opened her eyes and, for the first time ever, made eye contact with me. It was almost as though the electric shock had passed straight through her to me.

"Emma, are you with us?" I asked, astounded.

"Where am I? What day is it?" she croaked, and then started coughing again.

The nurse offered her a cup of water, which she held in both hands and lifted to her lips. She gulped it down, then sat forwards, alert. The nurse looked at me and I looked at the nurse. Our eyes widened; my heart pounded.

"So…you've just had ECT, it's Wednesday and…here you are. What does it feel like?"

Emma looked around the room.

"By the way, my name is—"

"Yes, I know who you are. You realise this is not going to last."

"Why not?"

"This is just a fight-or-flight reaction because of the stress you have put me under. It will probably reactivate the virus in my body and I'll end up worse off."

That sounded familiar.

"But you're speaking, you're moving, you can swallow. Isn't that great?"

"Yes, but it doesn't feel like it's really me, and anyway, I'll pay for it later." She arched her back and placed her hand above her hip, wincing with pain.

"It's good to talk, though," I ventured.

"I suppose so."

"Of course you are going to feel a bit stiff and weak. You've been flat on your back for over a year! I understand that you are worried that you may have a virus affecting your nervous system and that if you use up too much energy now, it might cause further damage. But what if we test out an alternative idea: that the virus was cleared from your body a long time ago and now you just need to gradually get moving again and to kind of get reconnected with your body."

"That's crap!"

"Think about it."

The nurse intervened. "Let's get you back to the ward and you can carry on the conversation there. And Emma, see you on Friday."

Emma smiled and gave a royal wave.

She wasn't quite able to stand up, her legs were wobbly, but she set herself down on an ordinary wheelchair. The first person to greet Emma on the ward was Christiana in full cleaning regalia. She did a double-take: *Oh. My. God.* Snapping off her disposable gloves and apron, she pulled Emma towards her ample bosom, almost smothering her. Christiana was sobbing tears of joy. Then cupping Emma's face in both hands, she said, "Look at you now, you're so beautiful. Thank the Lord."

The staff phoned Charles, who was at work. He hadn't felt it necessary to come for the ECT since the first one. Come quick, they said, there's nothing wrong – just come quick. After clinic, I went back to the ward and popped my head round Emma's side-room door. She was sitting up in bed with her father and they were going through a photograph album, chatting softly, eating chocolates. Charles told me they had managed to get hold of Miranda who had just phoned but wasn't going to be able to visit. It was all rather emotional (he squeezed her hand). Speaking for them both, he said they were tired and that Emma needed to rest.

The report from the next day was that Emma had slept well. In the morning, she stayed in bed and ate some yoghurt for breakfast. Her father visited briefly. She spoke to the day staff and therapy team, who were simply amazed and hastily drew up a new rehabilitation programme based on gradual increase in activities but with plenty of room to discuss fears of relapse and avoidance of a 'boom-and-bust' cycle. She then asked to be left alone and subsequently, as the day wore on, seemed to sink back into her previous unresponsive state. I went back to my office, somewhat deflated but knowing that we were on the right track. I checked my emails. There was one from Charles. He had never emailed me before. The message was plain: Emma had told him the previous night that she did not wish to have further ECT and therefore the treatment should cease.

After seeking the advice of colleagues, I replied to Charles the next morning that Emma had not raised any objections to me or any other member of staff, and today she is unable to communicate. I said the treatment was legally sanctioned and would go ahead. I offered to meet him again to discuss the matter that evening.

It was Friday, another ECT day; session number six. It proceeded as before. Again, miraculously, Emma woke up, immediately making eye contact as soon as she came round, and was eager to engage in debate. This time I had some of the therapy team by my side in the ECT suite so that they could witness the transformation and ask their own questions.

"So here we are again," was Emma's opening gambit.

"Indeed. First, is it true that you told your father that you didn't want any more ECT?"

"I told him it wasn't going to work. It was just a stress response."

"That's not the same thing."

"You can do what you want. It's not up to me. I have no control."

One of the therapists took over. "Emma, listen, if you really want the ECT to stop, tell us now but at least give a reason."

"There's no point discussing it. Didn't you know there's no such thing as free will? We're just machines. Please lay me flat." She smiled, turned her head away and closed her eyes.

Later, the physiotherapist, occupational therapist and I went to see Emma. She had managed to take a few steps with support from a person on either side – another momentous landmark. The therapists hoped they could agree on some goals to do with getting up, washing, feeding, toileting and so forth. They had a long chat, but the main thrust of it was Emma giving reasons why she couldn't do the activities, citing predicted bad effects it would have on her physical health. They did manage to elicit some preferences: tea *without* milk; not to be plonked in front of the TV during the day; therapists to come and see her at set times and not to keep 'popping in'; to ask her dad to bring in certain items of clothing and her hairbrush; if people insisted on having the radio on, could it be Radio 4 (news and current affairs) and not Radio 2 (easy listening). I asked whether we should still talk to her when she herself was unable to speak. She said, non-committal, she didn't mind. What about music; rather than Radio 2, what kind of stuff did she like?

"Silent music."

***

After Charles finished seeing Emma, he came to the interview room. He was looking pale and drawn.

"How was she?" I asked.

"Fine. She told me she had a lot of meetings today, so I didn't want to push her."

"But you would have preferred it if she had not had ECT and that no one would have been able to talk to her…"

"It's not a case of my preference but what Emma wants."

I composed myself. "It's just that I was struck by Christiana, one of our healthcare assistants, who has known Emma for, oh about three months. She was literally in tears when she saw Emma on Wednesday. While you, her father, sends me a curt email saying we should discontinue ECT, the only treatment that has given her a voice for the first time in about a year. You don't think that's…a bit odd?"

"Well, I apologise if it was curt. I appreciate you and the staff here are trying to do what you think is best for Emma. Make no mistake…I cherish every moment I have with her because I fear it may not last."

We stared at each other.

"By the way, I won't be visiting for a while. I need to go into hospital for some tests. Hopefully nothing serious."

I said I was sorry to hear about that and showed him out.

***

We applied for, and were granted, permission to give another tranche of six ECTs. A pattern emerged. In the lead-up to each session, Emma was the same: tremulous but silent and unresponsive. The effect was also the same: as soon as Emma came round from the GA, she would make eye contact and engage in conversation – albeit at times elliptical and enigmatic – but the duration of effect became progressively shorter.

Treatment eight was unusual. It was a substitute anaesthetist. After the intravenous anaesthetic was given, Emma's heart rate shot up and she became hot and flushed, so ECT was withheld. This was clearly an allergic reaction and it transpired that a different anaesthetic agent had been used. Emma did not speak at all or show any awareness after what was essentially 'sham ECT'. After treatment number nine, she spoke again, saying a few words, and then slipped into what looked like sleep. Later, she would open her eyes but look straight ahead and make no effort to communicate. After treatment ten, she said just one "hello"; treatment eleven, nothing; treatment twelve, again, nothing. One change that was maintained before and after the treatment was her ability to tolerate sitting and even standing up.

We did not propose any more ECT. The physiotherapists were pleased with Emma's increased mobility, which meant that she was not going to be at high risk of bedsores or pneumonia. Others and I spent long sessions talking to her, picking up on things she had said, trying to clarify them. What did she mean by not having free will? Was this her experience or some philosophy-of-mind throwaway she had heard on Radio 4? Was it evidence of psychosis? We gave her positive health messages on viral infections and immunity as well as on the importance of activity for joints and muscles. It made no tangible impact.

None of the staff missed having Charles around, but one evening, over two months after I'd last spoken to him, he turned up out of the blue. According to the night staff, he looked terrible. He had lost about two stones. His hair had thinned and his complexion was sallow. He told them that he had come to say goodbye to Emma. His cancer had come back and he was going into a hospice. He only had a couple of weeks left.

***

Getting Emma to the funeral was a logistical challenge requiring ambulances, ramps, wheelchairs and plenty of people to assist. We couldn't determine if she wanted to go but decided we should assume she did. A few old friends turned up. They spoke of Charles's public-spiritedness, his sense of duty and the unbearable stress he had endured (no doubt triggering the cancer relapse) from his daughter's condition and the unspeakable maltreatment she had suffered at the hands of psychiatry. Emma, positioned at the back of the hall, gave no indication that she was aware of the proceedings going on around her.

Later, the ward manager recalled that in previous situations where there was a highly enmeshed relationship between a parent and grown-up child with a severe mental disorder, the parent's death had sometimes heralded a new lease of life for the son or daughter. "Where there's death there's hope," he quipped, straining to lift the gloom.

***

Years later, Emma remains in precisely the same state. Why? Perhaps she is pining for her mother; she was brainwashed by her father, whom she loves or hates; she has a rare form of ECT-responsive catatonia or depression; she's got a chronic viral infection of the brain that biomedicine doesn't recognise; she has a brain disease invisible to the latest scanners; she's acting according to firmly held but erroneous illness beliefs; she's protesting; she's mad…

One clue, though it's hardly an explanation, comes from a magazine article on a Swedish persistent refusal case, or as they call it 'resignation' case, by *New Yorker* journalist Rachel Aviv.[20] It tells the story of Georgi who came from Russia at the age of five years with his family seeking asylum from religious persecution. They fought for six years to remain. When it seemed like their application had been rejected, Georgi developed the condition, sinking into an unresponsive, passive state for nearly a year. Finally, the family won their appeal and, slowly over a period of weeks, Georgi started to recover, initially just opening his eyes but later eating, drinking, talking and moving normally. When asked about his experience, looking back he said it started as a kind of protest: why would he go to school if he wasn't going to be able to live and work in the country? The protest then seemed to take on 'a momentum of its own' with his will seemingly draining away.

As for why Emma is in such a state? The truth is, nobody knows.

7

We Are Family

A family meal at Pizza Express had to be planned like a military operation.

> Step one: phone ahead to reserve a table for four (near the exit) at precisely 18.00 (not too busy).

> Step two: drop off mum at 17.59; place order including one pepperoni, large Coke (no ice), chocolate brownie.

> Step three: dad to circle around the block with Leo (age eleven years) and Christopher (age fifteen years) in back of car, until phone pings to signal order has arrived.

> Step four: return to restaurant, park, take seats, eat quickly, leave cash (including generous tip), exit together.

The family had learned through bitter experience that this was the only way to have any sort of evening out without causing a massive scene. Leo simply couldn't wait quietly at the table until the food arrived, or it wasn't the right thing, or there were too many people making a noise. He would start getting agitated, shouting "pepperoni Coke no ice" again and again. The situation would quickly escalate until he was punching himself in the forehead with both fists and wailing. People would stare, shake their heads, some sympathetically and others tutting, "disgraceful!"

Leo had autism; not autistic spectrum disorder, *proper* autism. It is a persistent and severe neurodevelopmental disorder which affects both the brain's structure and its function, particularly social behaviour and communication. It probably has a genetic origin, but we don't know exactly. Going to the cinema was not even worth thinking about. None of their friends invited them round and pizza seemed to be the only thing that Leo liked. The system worked and it got them out of the house, which was nice for Christopher.

The contrast with Christopher made Leo's disability even more stark, especially when it came to the usual milestones of growing up. First smile, first steps, first words – Leo had been way behind Christopher. He was diagnosed around the age of three or four years and had been going to a special school. The weekends and evenings were tough. The boys' father was a secondary-school teacher with head-of-department responsibilities; the mother, a nurse who often worked shifts. Christopher had a good way with Leo. He was very patient and relaxed and knew Leo's routines. They would play computer games, or watch videos, not together exactly but in the same room.

Christopher never complained, but there were times when he would seem withdrawn. Although he was well above average academically and good at sports – he was big for his age and played in goal for the school football team – he sometimes skipped school and wandered around the nearby common. Other boys got him to buy them cigarettes and some of the older ones pressured him to buy alcohol with a fake ID. He himself started smoking, which was stupid because he occasionally suffered from asthma. Worst of all, he started taking money out of his mother's purse to buy cigarettes.

One Friday he arranged to go to the cinema with some mates from school. Dad was away visiting his brother up north for a few days. His mum said she would be back early from the morning shift, so there should be no problem looking after Leo. However, she called around 5 p.m. to say she was having to stay on because they were short-staffed at the hospital.

"But I've arranged to go out tonight – for once!"

"I'm sorry, it's one of those things. I'll be home about nine. And stop being selfish," said his mother, impatiently. She wasn't exactly having a good day either.

Christopher fumed, went to his bedroom and slammed the door shut, ignoring Leo's request for something to eat. The boys' mother arrived home just after nine, as promised, to find Leo whimpering by the entrance. Christopher, who had been waiting in the hall in his anorak, was gone before she even had a chance to apologise.

The house rule was that Christopher had to be back home by 10 p.m. It passed 11 p.m. and his mother was starting to worry. Then midnight. He wasn't answering his phone. She didn't know what to do. Part of her wanted to call the police, but he was probably just hanging around the common.

It was after 1 a.m. when he stumbled in the front door and headed upstairs. He was dishevelled, his shoes muddy and you could smell the booze coming off him. He went straight to the bathroom without responding to his mother's questions and vomited down the toilet.

On the Sunday evening, both parents were home and confronted him. He was going off the rails and they were not going to sit back and let it happen. Why had he been missing school – had he forgotten that he had exams next year? Had he been stealing money? Christopher became extremely upset, crying and shouting as he protested his innocence, and he started shaking uncontrollably. Leo, meanwhile, cowered in the corner. The sanctions were tough. He was grounded. No way was Christopher going to be allowed to go on the special regional schools' football tour to Amsterdam at half-term.

The next morning, Christopher was reluctant to get ready for school. He was coughing and his breathing was wheezy. He was still shaking. His mum took pity on him. He could well have got a chest infection being out all night in the cold. She phoned the school to say he wouldn't be coming in that day. In fact, he didn't make it to school the whole week.

***

Christopher's mum took him to the doctor, who thought he probably did have a chest infection and prescribed antibiotics. He was breathing heavily, but it didn't seem like asthma. The shaking was a bit odd and a concern. Christopher's right arm shook from side to side in a coarse, irregular manner. It was very variable. Sometimes it stopped, especially when he was distracted, and even when active it didn't seem to interfere with dressing and eating. The doctor wondered whether the lad was using his asthma inhaler too much as that could cause a tremor, though it looked more like he was hyperventilating.

A week later, he finished the antibiotics. His breathing was better, but the shaking was still there. In fact, Christopher now started to complain that his right arm was weak and maybe his right leg too. The doctor examined him and couldn't find any abnormalities. His arms seemed equally strong when he was asked to hold them out in front of him while the doctor tried to push them down, but the right arm would all of a sudden give way and flop down to the side. The reflexes were normal and the same on both sides, suggesting that the nerves coming from his brain and down the spinal cord were intact.

The family oscillated between concern and annoyance. Had they been too harsh on Christopher? Or maybe he was just putting on an act? It was all very unsatisfactory and he wasn't explaining himself. They thought it would blow over and that 'making a fuss' would just exacerbate the problem; however, things were not improving. Eventually, he was referred to a paediatrician at the local hospital. She was both concerned and confounded. His neurological symptoms seemed to be progressing – he was now walking with a pronounced limp – but while the shaking did not resemble anything she knew about, it could be a rare movement disorder like childhood chorea (from the Greek verb 'to dance'). He was missing lots of school. She decided to admit him to hospital for some investigations. This would include blood tests, a brain scan and X-rays of the spine, and a lumbar puncture (LP) to obtain a sample of cerebrospinal fluid (CSF) which could be examined primarily for evidence of inflammation inside the nervous system.

By the time he was admitted, Christopher was walking with a Zimmer frame and needed help dressing and washing. His mum and dad had been providing the extra care, consumed with guilt that they had overreacted to their son's naughty but hardly outrageous behaviour. They were ashamed and, as public servants, they were determined that their 'stupidity' would not burden the state. They would bear the consequences of their actions.

The brain scan and X-rays were normal, which was hugely reassuring; that meant there was no tumour and nothing pressing on the spinal cord. Then came the LP, a routine procedure but one that causes discomfort for the patient and requires some skill on the part of the doctor. The patient, stripped to their underpants, lies on the examination couch on their left side, curled up in a tight ball. The skin is swabbed with an antiseptic. The nurse will drape the lower back with a sterile sheet with a square hole in the middle which is positioned over the lumbar spine. The doctor sits on a stool behind the patient and feels their way down the spine to find the shallow dip between the last two vertebrae of the lumbar spine just above the pelvis. A tiny area is injected with local anaesthetic; sometimes the patient will flinch slightly, but the pain is minimal. Then the doctor is handed the LP needle. He or she checks the target area again and says something along the lines of, "You're going to feel a bit of pushing now…" The needle should then slide in smoothly, avoiding any bony obstacle. The inner core of the needle is withdrawn and, all being well, after a couple of seconds the first drop of CSF, the colour and consistency of white wine, should emerge pleasingly out of the end of the needle and drip gently into the specimen bottles held below, to be sent to the laboratory.

Psychiatrists don't do these kinds of procedures. When I was a junior doctor working in neurology I used to enjoy doing LPs and considered myself an expert. On one occasion I was told by my consultant to do an LP on a man in his forties who had been admitted with a sudden, severe headache and who was now a little drowsy and had a stiff neck. The CT scan didn't show very much and the routine at the time was to do an LP to check if he had an aneurysm or meningitis. Surrounded by student nurses, I played to the gallery. Having put in the local anaesthetic, I took the LP needle and, for the benefit of my audience, explained what I was about to do. At that moment the patient let out a thundering and prolonged fart. "Ex-cuse me!" I retorted with high-camp indignation. The nurses giggled. It took a few seconds to dawn on me that the patient had just made his last sound. The aneurysm was presumably about to give at any moment and, perhaps as the patient braced himself for the needle, it burst. I don't believe I caused him to die, but I can't get over the shame of my vain and crass behaviour. I stopped doing them after that.

***

For his LP, Christopher was agitated and was finding it difficult to lie still. His arm was shaking. He was muscly and a little overweight, so it was hard to find the right spot between the vertebrae where the needle should go. When the local anaesthetic needle (no bigger than a pin) went in, his body lurched forwards, almost falling off the couch. The junior doctor was not feeling confident. Tentatively he pushed the LP needle in – forgetting to warn Christopher. Christopher straightened up reflexively, making it much more difficult to pass the needle between the vertebrae. With the needle half in, the doctor and assisting nurse tried to get Christopher back in position, asking him to try to keep still.

The doctor pushed the needle further, but it hit some bone. Christopher groaned. The needle was pulled out. A bead of blood oozed from the puncture site. The nurse tried to reassure Christopher that he was doing well; it didn't quite work that time, but they would have another go in a minute. And so they did. It was even worse. Christopher was fidgeting even before the doctor made his move. More local anaesthetic was injected. The LP needle seemed to go in. The doctor pulled back the inner core and waited. No fluid. They abandoned the procedure. The doctor then called the registrar, his senior colleague who agreed to stop by later that day to repeat the procedure. Even the registrar, who had probably done a hundred LPs in his time, took two tries but eventually succeeded. It was a 'traumatic tap', meaning the fluid was contaminated with blood from the tissues penetrated by the needle on the way in, which is just about acceptable, though not ideal, for analysis. Everyone was relieved, except Christopher. The doctor told him how well he had done and that the worst was over, but he was a quivering wreck.

Christopher's whole body was shaking now. Waxing and waning, it went on for hours. He was also complaining of severe pain in his back and said that he could not move either of his legs. The junior doctor was called to see him, anxious that it might be a complication of the LP. The only way something like this could have happened, he thought, was if there had been a tumour in the brain. That could have caused pressure to build inside the skull and, when the pressure had been released with the puncture, the brain would have been forced downwards against the skull, causing irreparable damage. But that was impossible because the CT scan, which was done prior to the LP precisely to avoid such a complication, was completely clear.

An emergency EEG was ordered just in case the shaking was due to some kind of epileptic seizure. The tracing showed normal brain activity, but this was drowned out by Christopher's agitation ('muscle contraction artefact'). The registrar was also called and examined Christopher himself, again worried that he had done something wrong. He couldn't explain Christopher's reaction other than that it was a psychological consequence of the fear evoked by the LP, heightened by the repetition and pain. But this was not really an adequate explanation of the fact that he had suddenly lost the use of his legs. There was some discernible movement and Christopher could still sit himself up and manoeuvre himself in the bed, which he couldn't have done if his legs were totally paralysed.

The consultant reviewed Christopher the next day and carried out a full examination. She could not explain the deterioration in his condition through any physical mecha-nism. The CSF analysis from the LP came back normal. A clini-cal psychologist was called in who saw Christopher for a number of sessions on his own and with the family. He contacted the school and spoke to the GP. It took a few weeks, but the psychologist compiled a detailed report which proposed that Christopher was suffering from what he called a 'conver-sion disorder', which he explained had occurred as a result, at least in part, of psychological conflict manifesting as a neuro-logical disability. The report speculated that it was all part of Christopher's difficulty adjusting to his circumstances: resent-ment of the attention Leo was getting; difficulty living up to his parents' expectations; unhappiness at school; and health concerns (i.e. asthma and becoming overweight). This had come to a head on that fateful Friday night and Christopher had 'learned', perhaps unconsciously, that he could avoid the pressures of family and school and bullying by being ill. Then there was the LP. While none of these factors are in themselves extraordinary, they add up, in the psychologist's view, to a suffi-cient cause of Christopher's sudden disablement; all the more so when combined with Christopher's temperament, which he judged to be anxious, and with the LP, which had been fright-ening and 'traumatic' (in the psychological as well as the physi-cal sense). This had led to 'decompensation' and 'regression' to an earlier childlike state of dependence. The recommendation was for a full course of individual psychotherapy combined with physiotherapy and gradual rehabilitation. The prognosis for conversion disorder in a young person, diagnosed and treated early, was thought to be good.[1]

Christopher remained in the hospital's neurorehabilitation unit for eighteen months without improvement; in fact, he deteriorated to the point that he lost all useful function in both of his hands and arms as well as his legs. He was bedbound, effectively paralysed from the neck down. Although he retained bowel and bladder sensation, he had to be lifted onto the toilet. He adopted a method of using a computer by holding a thin plastic stick between his teeth and tapping the keyboard with it. His dad tried to maintain his schooling by bringing his textbooks and assignments, but it was hopeless. He did not take his exams.

Christopher did not show any obvious signs of depression. He expressed frustration at his predicament but cooperated with the physiotherapists who were eventually reduced to simply massaging his limbs and moving them passively to prevent the muscle tendons and joints becoming stiff. It was at this point that Christopher was referred to our neuropsychiatry unit.

***

We were taking more and more patients with conversion disorders, or functional neurological disorders as they were becoming known. The term 'conversion' dates back to the nineteenth century, when it was thought that emotional conflict which could not be articulated was 'converted' into a physical symptom. Sigmund Freud and Josef Breuer put this on the intellectual map with their *Studies on Hysteria*, published in 1895, using even older terminology harking back to the ancient Greeks and their notions of the uterus (*hustera*) wandering around the body disrupting internal organs. It soon became clear that this was not a condition exclusive to women, nor was it instantly cured by bringing the unconscious conflict to the surface through psychoanalysis or hypnosis. Nevertheless, the stories behind those cases were captivating and compelling.

The link between conversion and sex or sexual abuse, which so scandalised *fin de siècle* Vienna, is now accepted as a key factor in many cases, though certainly not all.[2] Similarly, the notion that the mind – ideas, fears, fantasies, beliefs, conflicts and that catch-all 'stress' – could play out via the body, outside clearly intended actions, stubbornly resists dismissal. The conversion hypothesis, especially when supported by the temporal order of cause and effect as in Christopher's case, can indeed be compelling,[3] although – here comes a health warning – just because a case sounds compelling, fulfils a satisfying narrative arc and makes sense of the otherwise inexplicable, that doesn't mean it's true.

Our notions of what a 'real' illness is, and what role and responsibilities the ill person has or is excused from by society, have given rise to the constructs of 'the sick role' and 'illness behaviour'.[4]

On top of this, advances in medical diagnostics mean that practitioners can be comfortable deeming the patient to have the appearance of a neurological disorder without the physical evidence to support it, although there is, for some, the nagging doubt that it is just a matter of time until, with some new technology, such evidence will be uncovered.

Into this quagmire of uncertainty steps the neuropsychiatrist, anchored by the important bedrock of the 'biopsychosocial' approach. Each strand, each perspective (biological, psychological and social), should be examined with an open mind and the evidence considered. In a given disorder, one or other perspective may carry more weight, but it's rare that there are no relevant or illuminating contributions from each of the biological, psychological or social realms. The psychiatrist must remain undogmatic and open to each of these different intellectual, evidence-based traditions, as well as leaving room for uncertainty.

In Christopher's case, there was a complication: the district health authority did not want to approve the referral. Not understanding the need for specialist input, they wondered why their local clinical teams couldn't do the necessary work. Why should their valuable resources leak out of the borough to fund a tertiary centre, the equivalent, in their minds, of a sort of metropolitan elite? There was also the plainly artificial demarcation between services for minors and adults. No, they would rather institute a 'comprehensive care package' and look after the patient in his own home. This seemed to undermine the principles of a *National* Health Service, but that is how the system worked then and to some extent still does, with a split between commissioners and providers brought in to improve 'efficiency'.

***

Christopher was sent home. The modest suburban semi where he lived would need extensive modifications, a proper hospital bed, full-body hoists, adapted shower and toilet facilities, wheelchair access, the lot. And what about Leo? He would probably need more care too. His parents were in a state of quiet desperation. They would probably need to consider giving up work or drastically reducing their hours. The tragedy was that Christopher's condition was treatable, possibly even curable. I could not let this go.

I wrote a long letter to the director and commissioner of Mental Health Services, setting out the reasons why the local services simply did not have the relevant expertise or facilities to take on such a case: Christopher needed urgent inpatient neuropsychiatric rehabilitation. I poured all of my righteous anger into it as I explained the likely knock-on effects on the rest of the family and how this would be extremely costly: day care for Leo, visits at least four times a day from a bank of carers, possibly the loss of an experienced nurse from the NHS, and the giving out of benefits and allowances. I added that his condition was much more likely to respond to treatment if it was given as early as possible. As I made these arguments I suspected they were futile. For a start, all these new costs would come out of someone else's budget. I was also advised that I would not be seen as an impartial NHS clinician seeking to steer a complex patient towards the right therapy but as a service provider with a 'conflict of interests'.

I never received a reply. I tried a different tack: if they wouldn't listen to me, then surely they would listen to 'one of their own', the local general practitioner faced with coordinating the care package, knowing how inadequate it would be. The GP did not need any persuasion and started to lobby on behalf of Christopher and his family. He did confide in me that while mum and dad were in favour of specialist help, they were somewhat passive and declined to get involved in what amounted to a campaign. It seemed that they blamed themselves and felt that it was their fate to accept all that life threw at them. They were not, as they often said, the sort of people to make a fuss.

***

Inevitably I had to move on, and my attention turned to another patient, Amy. She had very little recollection of how she ended up in casualty; her husband, Mark, told her that she'd had a fit. She had been feeling 'off' that day and had a pounding headache. Jade, her seven-year-old daughter, had come home from school with her friend and the friend's mum to find Amy spreadeagled on the kitchen floor. They rushed over to her. She was awake but drowsy. There was a tiny trickle of blood down the side of her mouth from where she had bitten her tongue. They called an ambulance and then phoned Mark who left work immediately to meet them at the hospital. It turned out that she'd had another fit in the ambulance. The paramedics were sure it was an epileptic seizure. It had all the hallmarks, starting with some twitching on the right side of her body, her head turning to the left, eyes wide open, followed by really strong tensing of all the muscles in the body, clenching of the jaw and rhythmic jerking for about thirty to forty seconds, dying away with the odd single jerk, leaving her floppy and asleep for a minute or two before coming round.

She had not had epilepsy as a child and, at age forty-two, there was likely to be an underlying cause. Looking back on it, for a couple of months she had been having headaches a lot more than usual. She had no other symptoms except that sometimes she just could not find the right word for something, but then, we all get that sometimes, don't we? A CT scan done that evening showed a round craggy mass, a brain tumour about the size of a golf ball in her left frontal lobe. It looked like a fairly high-grade astrocytoma,[5] meaning it was likely to grow and invade the surrounding brain tissue over the coming months.

The consultant met Amy and Mark on the neurosurgical ward a few days later. It was not good news, but there were plenty of treatments available. First, they would put her on steroids to reduce the swelling around the tumour, which would stop the headaches, and they would start her on anti-convulsant medication. She would be offered radiotherapy and possibly chemotherapy, but this would be discussed with the oncology team. She was otherwise well: all the tests had come back clear and there was no sign of cancer anywhere else in her body. They would really have liked to take a biopsy of the tumour to find out more about the kind of tissue it contained, but because of its position, near the speech area of the brain, it wasn't an option.

It was all pretty devastating, but they were thankful for the calm and reassuring manner in which the surgeon had spoken to them and for him seeming to be quite optimistic. He tried to duck Mark's obvious 'how long?' question by saying that it was a bit early for all of that and, besides, some people survive for many, many years. They took this to mean it could be *months*. They explained to Jade that mummy was sick but that she was going to be OK. They had to look after each other. They were a strong family and loved each other very much. They would get through it. There were lots of tears and hugs.

***

About three months later, Amy found herself back on the neurosurgical ward. The treatment had been going well, but lately she'd started having seizures again, mostly just small ones where her right arm would jerk and she'd feel spaced out. Increasing the anticonvulsants had probably helped, but then she'd had a really bad run with one seizure, leading to another, and another with no respite. Perhaps unsurprisingly, she was feeling low.

When I saw her on the ward she was sat up in bed, her face tear-stained and puffy due to the steroids. She was pleased to talk. It was boring being in hospital waiting for tests and specialist opinions. She was witty, self-deprecating and brave. I warmed to her. She spoke about Jade and Mark, whose pictures surrounded her bedside, and how they were all hoping to go to Disneyland soon. I didn't think she was depressed or needed any more medication, but rather she was facing her future and trying to deal with it. I was about to leave when she started crying. It wasn't a normal cry; she was clenching her teeth and groaning, making a low-pitched guttural sound.

"Amy, are you OK? What's happening?"

She didn't respond but stared ahead, clutching her knees against her chest, rocking back and forth. One of the nurses stepped over to see what was happening.

"She's having another one of her fits," the nurse said as she pulled the curtain round.

Now the groaning became louder and turned into a prolonged wail. The rocking became more insistent, but there was no jerking or shaking. I motioned to the nurse to stand by. It continued for about three minutes and then the rocking slowed down and the wailing softened. Amy seemed to be saying "no, no, no" in time with the rocking, tears still streaming down her face. I held her hand.

"It's OK Amy, can you hear me? You're not having a seizure, you are upset and must be frightened. Let it pass; it's over now…"

Amy opened her eyes and nodded in response, then lay back on her pillow. The nurse took over, mopping Amy's face with a tissue, and put an arm around her, consoling her. The whole episode lasted about ten minutes.

"What happened?" asked Amy, seemingly perplexed. "Was it a fit?"

I explained to both Amy and the nurse that these were 'functional seizures'. Sometimes people feel overwhelmed by emotions – sadness, fear, it could be anything – and, a bit like a safety valve, the mind just switches off and the body just does its own thing. We call it dissociation. It is especially likely to occur if you're feeling spaced out anyway due to medication or fatigue, and actually, it is not that uncommon in people who have epileptic seizures as well.[6]

I stayed a while with Amy as she collected herself and we spoke more about what had happened.

"It's true I am feeling overwhelmed. A lot has been happening recently. You wouldn't believe it. And you know my biggest fear? It's that I won't be around to protect Jade." She started to cry all over again.

I nodded and tried to think of something useful to say. Suddenly it struck me what she had said. "Protect Jade from what?"

There was a long pause. Amy looked towards the curtains, indicating that we needed privacy.

"I've never spoken to anyone about this before, even Mark. When I was seven, Jade's age now, I was…abused, sexually." She fought back more tears. "It was the summer holidays. My cousin Bob came round one morning. He was twelve at the time. I had got a new cassette recorder for my birthday. Bob had some tapes and my mum said, 'Why don't you go up to Jade's bedroom and listen to music, she would love that'. We sat on the bed, lying back, listing to pop songs, then suddenly he pushed his hand under my nightie. I had no idea what was going on. It happened again and again throughout the holidays. My mum and Bob's dad, Uncle Harry, were close and they only lived round the corner. They were always popping round. It went on for years. Bob was threatening. He said if I ever told anyone, they wouldn't believe me and would put me in a home. Year after year it went on, until he was fifteen and I must have been about eleven. One day he met me after school, took me to a wood and raped me. I ran home and told my mum what had happened. She told me I had been stupid, that he was only a boy and I must have led him on. We never spoke about it again. What she said to Uncle Harry and Bob I never knew, but they stopped coming round."

It was an awful account, but sadly I had heard similar tales before.[7] Amy seemed to be relieved that she had finally spoken about it. She knew that it wasn't really her fault, even if she still struggled to understand it. Not being consoled at the time still stung. Uncle Harry had been going through a divorce, so it was a difficult time for Bob. They were just kids, but on the other hand, the age gap was significant. There was a large power imbalance, and by fifteen he must've known that what he was doing was wrong. As for her mum, that was simply what her generation was like. Her own upbringing was harsh: she was one of seven, they were poor and there wasn't much affection.

We arranged for Amy to have some sessions in the outpatient clinic after she went home. I was confident we could help her manage the functional seizures and said we needed to work closely with the neurosurgeons regarding her anticonvulsants and tumour treatment. I said she should consider telling Mark.

Before we parted, I recalled another comment she made about there being a lot happening. What did she mean? She explained that after years of avoiding Uncle Harry, out of the blue they had received an invitation – to Bob's wedding. Mark thought it would be a great day out. Amy's mum thought they should all go. The wedding was last weekend. She had had a couple of seizures that morning so they couldn't make it anyway.[8]

***

Meanwhile, back on our neuropsychiatry unit, we were expecting a new admission. Unbelievably it had taken another full year before finally, it was agreed that Christopher (now eighteen) could be admitted 'for a trial period'. Once settled, members of the multidisciplinary team carried out their assessments.[9] Christopher was one of the most disabled people we had ever been asked to treat. Everyone found him to be a polite, friendly, serious young man. His mum and dad were similar: grateful and deferential. He appeared to be as mystified as all of us regarding his condition. He accepted that all his tests and scans were normal, but somehow that didn't help. The sight of him, a strong-looking, thick-set young man over six feet tall, laboriously tapping at his computer with the tool between his teeth in order to send emails and search the internet – like someone with paraplegia due to a broken neck – was shocking. And after such a long delay, was he even treatable?

After interviewing Christopher and going through many of the issues raised in the clinical psychologist's report, I thought it would be instructive to examine him physically myself. He lay on his back in the bed propped up by pillows. I asked him to raise his right leg: there was barely a flicker of movement. I then asked him to push down on the bed with his right heel, which I cupped in my hand: there was no power at all. Next I asked him to raise his left leg: this time with some effort, Christopher's leg rose slowly off the bed, wobbled for a few seconds, then wilted back down. I asked him to do it again, placing my left hand on top of his left shin, and told him to push against me. At the same time I slipped my right hand surreptitiously under his right heel as before: the left leg came up.

"Good, well done, hold it there."

As he did this I could feel some tension in the previously paralysed right leg. As I tried to lift it up from the heel, there was obvious contraction in the muscles working against me. The pushing stopped and he exhaled with relief.

"You see what happened just then? When you were concentrating on lifting your left leg, your right leg seemed to find some strength."

Christopher was flummoxed.

"You see, it's a natural reflex. When you raise one leg, the other automatically pushes down to maintain balance. But when you try to do it consciously, nothing happens."

"But I really was trying!"

"I know. I'm showing you that what you have is functional paralysis. That means the messages are not getting through from your brain to your muscles. I'm not sure why. The important thing is that the connections are still there and they do work but you have to sort of do it indirectly. But it's good news. The structure, the nerves – the body's own wiring – are intact, and there's no permanent physical damage."[10]

I could see that Christopher was engaged and understood the implications. It was possible that he could progress, but it was a lot to take in all at once.

"You know what happens to sportsmen sometimes, even the best ones. They choke. You were a goalie. You know what can happen when there's a penalty kick. The striker steps up and all he has to do is hit it from twelve yards with the whole goal to aim at…"

"Yeah, sometimes they completely scuff it. It's crazy."

"When we are really stressed and self-conscious, and maybe trying too hard, actions that usually happen almost on their own, like walking, kicking a ball, suddenly seem…really complicated. But if we keep calm, don't think about it and just let it happen, it usually does."

People who have one-sided weakness or struggle to walk normally can sometimes really take off from this point. Skilled physiotherapists, like Glenn Nielsen working in London, have come up with a number of ingenious techniques to help patients overcome functional neurological disorders.[11] For example, they will get them to do things like walk backwards so that the intense and futile effort that they were putting into their gait, one laborious step after another, is undermined and they suddenly find that walking backwards 'without thinking' is easier than walking forwards.[12] It seems that with functional neurological disorders, paradoxically, the less you try, the easier it gets. But Christopher was too profoundly impaired. We needed to get a little bit more movement in his limbs to have something to build on.

Part of the diagnostic testing for neuromuscular disorders is transcranial magnetic stimulation (TMS). This involves a magnetic coil, made into a paddle like a small ping-pong bat, through which a pulse of electric current is passed. This induces a magnetic field for a fraction of a second. If the paddle is placed over the correct part of the brain's motor cortex where signals to move the limbs originate, or lower down their path like the spinal cord, or nerve roots as they exit the spine, this can induce a harmless current which, when conducted through nerves, results in a twitch in the connected muscle group. The clinical neurophysiologist can record even microscopic contractions by inserting into the muscle a fine needle connected to an amplifier and recording device. From this, they can tell if the pattern of firing is normal and the muscle itself is healthy. He or she can also measure the time in milliseconds between the stimulation coming from the magnetic coil and the contraction to determine if the speed of nerve condition is normal or slowed down. It's just like an electrician testing a circuit.

Christopher was wheeled into the neurophysiology testing lab. After some preliminary calibration to set the thresholds on the machine, the neurophysiologist got to work. Placing the paddle mostly around the neck and recording from Christopher's calves, various clicks, beeps and crackles emanated from the equipment. Reading the numbers off an LED screen, he said that all the conduction times were within normal limits and the muscles were contracting when induced to do so. All that was reassuring and we repeated the message that the connections were intact but that "we just needed to get the current flowing again." Christopher was unimpressed. We thought we would try something a bit different. Instead of using the minimum stimulus required to produce a twitch, why not make it a bit stronger? We cranked up the machine, put the paddle over the motor cortex and pressed the red button. There was the usual audible click, but this time it produced a visible jerk.

"Whoa! What was that?" said Christopher.

Another pulse. This time the paralysed right leg shot out.

"Hey, how did you do that?"

The same thing happened again.

Christopher shook his head. "That is amazing!"

Next we turned to the recording from the muscles. This was rigged up to a loudspeaker which emitted a series of clicks corresponding to each muscle-fibre contraction. You could easily turn up the volume. The normally taciturn neurophysiologist spoke to Christopher directly and said that having shown that those calf muscles were working, we would like to see him do it on his own. All eyes turned to the little green wire coming from the needle in Christopher's leg. Click. Click-click. Click, came the sound. "C'mon, you can do better than that," we urged. Click-click-click… The noise grew, the rhythm quickened. It was like one of those metal detectors coming upon a pile of buried coins. Buzzzzzzzz went the machine. "Brilliant!" we said in unison. True, the foot barely moved, it was a touch of theatre aided by turning the volume up to the maximum, but it made a real impression. Suddenly Christopher was getting some positive feedback from his efforts and with it came hope. He couldn't stop laughing. And for me, far from being the 'heart-sink' patient that Christopher might have been, from that day onward, I was sure he was going to be a therapeutic success.

The next session was in the gym with the physiotherapists. Christopher was held dangling from a hoist, over parallel bars. His feet barely touched the ground, but his hands naturally curled round the bars at waist level. He was lowered a few more millimetres. Reflexively, his legs straightened and some of his weight went through them. A stream of encouragement came from the physiotherapists as he tried to lift his better left leg to take his first tentative step.

Weeks passed and with each day there were incremental improvements in Christopher's abilities. The occupational therapist tackled the computer stick. She'd argued that we should take it away, as an experiment, to see if with his wrists placed on a foam support he couldn't turn the faintest flicker of movement in his fingers into a useful key press. Yes, he could; each little victory built on the previous one. The atmosphere changed. The clinical psychologist had her sessions and these were bearing fruit as well. Christopher was a good patient. He enjoyed the mechanistic understanding he was being given with its references to the brain and neuroscience. He felt he was being treated like an adult for the first time. They started talking about home life and future ambitions. He wanted to get his qualifications but thought he needed to leave home. He loved his parents and Leo, but they didn't see him as an adult. He needed to be independent.

After about four months, Christopher was getting around almost normally with a rather rakish walking stick and still improving. He was able to feed and dress himself and use a computer. He got tired at times, but everyone knew he would be OK. His parents were of course delighted. It was an amazing transformation.

I felt another letter coming on. I proposed to write again to the person in charge of approving referrals for specialist treatment, showing how unconscionable was their decision to deny a young lad the chance to be freed from incapacitating paralysis for, yes, four whole years. I would complain to the Care Quality Commission, the General Medical Council and the press until they apologised profusely to Christopher and his family. I put this idea to the family and they were less keen. Why dwell on the past? He's doing so well, so why jinx it? The local team were only trying to do their best. With hindsight, we all might have behaved differently, and no, they didn't want to make a fuss.

***

I saw Amy for a review in the clinic, with husband Mark. It was about a year after she was diagnosed with the brain tumour. She had gone noticeably downhill. She walked pushing a kind of trolley on wheels for stability. Her speech was halting, and she missed connecting words. Amy's brain tumour had destroyed the parts of the left frontal lobe responsible for expressive speech and for controlling the right side of the body. (More severe damage can reduce speech to just a few common words or even just parts of words.)

"Struggle…walking slow…speech, trying best…no fits, hurrah!" She made a thumbs-up sign.

Mark gently and tactfully tried to help. "Yes, it's been tough but could be a lot worse. We've had great support from the hospital and the Macmillan team, and have had some real quality time together as a family. It's been hard for Jade, but she's OK. Amy's mum has really stepped up and been amazing. We couldn't have done it without her."

Amy threw me a glance. I took this to mean she hadn't told him. How cruel it was that, not long after Amy was able to articulate her memories of abuse after years of silence, and the irreconcilable dilemmas that she found herself in, the ability to find the right words was denied her.[13]

We talked a while and it was taxing for her. There wasn't much for me to do. I wished them well and we said goodbye. Mark phoned the next day. They had parked the car by a meter just around the corner from the hospital. The appointment took longer than they had expected and, because of Amy's mobility problems, they'd ended up getting a parking ticket. He wondered if I could help, write a letter perhaps. Too right! I picked up the Dictaphone and out came a stream of exquisitely honed, controlled rage.

I heard nothing and forgot about it until six months later, when I received a handwritten letter from Mark. He thought I'd like to know that, against all expectation, they had received confirmation from the council saying that they had considered our appeal against the parking fine and had decided to award a full refund. That letter had done the trick. He thanked me for all I had done. He continued: "Amy passed away two weeks ago. We were all together at home, which is what she wanted, and she was very peaceful at the end."

***

The last time I saw Christopher was in the outpatient clinic. He came alone on public transport. It was wonderful to see him. He was physically impressive and rather handsome. He grinned broadly as he gave me an update. He was at college doing A levels, still living at home but looking to find a flat-share. There were some dips in his mood as he tried to come to terms with the wasted years, how his school friends were already going to university or jobs, and fears that he might slip back, but all that was manageable.

I asked him whether, looking back, he understood what had happened to him, what it felt like to be simply unable to move your own body. Alas, there was no revelation. Christopher said he just felt detached, "like it wasn't my body to move." It had all been baffling and strange. He recalled the lumbar puncture; he was scared witless. It felt like the doctors were shoving a dagger into his spinal cord until, all of a sudden, all feeling left him. When asked what he found most helpful, he was clear: the positive and accepting attitude of all the team; and an explanation for what was wrong with him that at least kind of made sense. And the TMS? Yes, that definitely made a difference; it had given him a tangible sign that he could recover.[14]

***

I often think of Amy and Christopher. They were so different and yet they had much in common. They both had functional

neurological disorders and any attempt to separate compo-
nents of their conditions into mental and physical would have
been doomed. Each of them provides an exemplary case
against a rigid form of mind–body dualism, which haunts
much of the clinical work in the area of neuropsychiatry, and
in favour of a richer kind of holism. I don't believe there is any
kind of spirit or life force apart from our material brains,
which leaves me open to the charge of reductionism. If my
years of practice have confirmed anything to me, it is that
everything in our mental life does come down to, can be
reduced to, the workings of our brains. But then, our brains
exist in an interconnected world of experience and moulding
influences. So the real challenge is finding the right level of
explanation along the biological, psychological and social
continuum.

Think of a great novel. How best to understand it? From a
distance, all books look the same. Under the microscope, all
we see is dots of pigment on cellulose. But somewhere between
the extremes, we find a tapestry of meanings woven into
language and culture. For some people, life can turn on a single
molecule disrupting the genetic code, or the misfiring of a
cluster of neurones; for others, there is no way to understand
or resolve life's dilemmas without considering, and perhaps
decoding, our shared history.

Science could do nothing to stop Amy's brain tumour growing, nor did it provide a useful readout of what was going on in
Christopher's mind. It didn't correct the past or provide an
alternative family life for either of them. For some of the scientific challenges, it may just be a matter of time. But, spanning

all these domains, there has always been a kind of medicine that can reach out across the abyss to find some level of understanding, that can restore faith, and every now and then can transform lives utterly.

Acknowledgements

I would like to thank all my colleagues, teachers, mentors, students and of course patients to whom I owe everything. I am especially grateful to Louis Appleby, Charles Geekie, Michael David, Andrew Hodgkiss, Eduardo Iacoponi, Sameer Jauhar, Nick Medford, Tim Nicholson and Ulrike Schmidt for commenting on draft chapters, and to 'Patrick', 'Victoria', 'Jennifer' and 'Christopher' for assenting to my drawing on their experiences.

I would also like to extend special gratitude to my editor, Alex Christofi, whose unstinting eye for detail and ear for resonance has elevated a series of case reports into something resembling an actual book.

In telling the stories contained in this volume, I have done my utmost to protect the anonymity of the people concerned. In all cases names, ages and sometimes genders and other identifying characteristics have been changed, as well as key facts, to ensure that individuals are so disguised as to be unrecognisable. Many stories are in fact amalgamations of several people and events. Nevertheless, I hope I have retained the essential 'truth' underlying these stories and have done justice to the lives and realities that underpin them. I trust that this will be seen as helpful and illuminating to people with similar problems or conditions, and that this justifies the use of cases drawn from real life.

Notes

Introduction

1   Bolton, D. and Gillett, G., *The Biopsychosocial Model of Health and Disease*. (Cham: Palgrave Pivot, 2019), pp. 1–145 (recently published critique and defence of the model from two clinician philosophers).

2   Jaspers, K., *General Psychopathology* (7th edn), trans. J. Hoenig and M.W. Hamilton (Baltimore: Johns Hopkins University Press, 1913/1997).

3   Laing, R.D., *The Divided Self*. Modern Classics. (London: Penguin Books, 2010) [first published as *The Divided Self: A Study of Sanity and Madness*. (London: Tavistock Publications, 1960)].

1. Dopamine

1   Fahn, S., 'The History of Dopamine and Levodopa in the Treatment of Parkinson's Disease', *Movement Disorders*, 23 (Suppl 3), 2008, pp. S497–508.

2   Howes, O.D., 'What the New Evidence Tells Us About Dopamine's Role in Schizophrenia', in *Schizophrenia: The Final Frontier – a Festschrift for Robin M. Murray*. eds A.S. David, S. Kapur and P. McGuffin (Hove East Sussex: Psychology Press, 2011), pp. 365–72.

3   Crow, T.J., Johnstone, E.C. and McClelland, H.A. 'The Coincidence of Schizophrenia and Parkinsonism: Some Neurochemical Implications', *Psychological Medicine*, 6, 1976, pp. 227–33.

4   The fact of the efficacy of clozapine is another blow to the dopamine hypothesis of schizophrenia, although not a fatal one. It does block

dopamine receptors but only very weakly. It is also known to affect a broad range of other neurotransmitter systems; hence, its relatively benign side-effect profile in terms of movement.

5   Rogers, J., Pollak, T., Blackman, G. and David, A.S. (2019) 'Catatonia and Immune Dysregulation: A Review'. [Online]. (http://dx.doi. org/10.1016/S2215-0366(19)30190-7). *Lancet Psychiatry* 6 (7). (Accessed 1 July 2019).

6   There are many neurological and psychiatric phenomena which benefit from an analysis using a cybernetic approach (see Spence, S.A., 'Alien Motor Phenomena: A Window on to Agency', *Cognitive Neuropsychiatry*, 7, 2002, pp. 211–20). Of course you have to start with the instruction or 'will' to move. A 'move' signal is then passed down towards the motor controller which in turn selects and switches on the relevant machinery. Information on the movement is then fed back to a 'comparator' so that adjustments can be made; for example, if the arm is about to under- or over-shoot, it can be corrected. The instructor ideally needs to be able to distinguish its own intended actions from those arising elsewhere; hence, each time an instruction is issued, it sends out a message to the comparator to expect an action, like a confirmation email when you book some tickets online, known technically as an efference copy. So if something takes hold of your arm and moves it this way or that, there is no efference copy; the 'system' therefore concludes that the movement is coming from outside, even without your seeing what's going on. Similarly, if an intention (with efference copy) to move is not followed by the sensation of movement (or feedback that movement is taking place), then clearly it's not a problem with the message itself but the message is not getting through. A person with Parkinson's disease may be unable to move or unable to execute anything like the movement they wish to perform. The intention is there; they can feel it because of the efference copy, and with that, a sense of effort, but it just doesn't happen. Conversely, if the person has a tremor (another key symptom of the disease), they know that it is not they themselves that is deliberately doing the movement, but rather that it is happening *to* them ("it's the Parkinson's that's doing it"). What may be the problem in passivity experiences is that the intention to move isn't followed by an efference copy (the confirmation email isn't sent or doesn't get through), so the person doesn't feel they own it; instead, it feels like someone else is in charge. Why is this different from the

tremor in Parkinson's disease? Perhaps in Parkinson's disease it is the actual machinery that is malfunctioning – disease has caused it to break down – but in passivity in schizophrenia the problem is happening 'higher up' in the system at the level of intention itself. The movement has all the hallmarks of an intended action, the sort of thing I might do or might have done before, it's just that on this occasion it lacks the sense of *me* doing it. I didn't get the email! The seat of the problem is in the efference-copy bit of the system – it's not working reliably – rather than in the execution of intended movement. Another explanation is that the problem lies not in the mechanisms of control but in attribution. This is our propensity to try to explain everything, particularly the unexpected. Depending on who we are, our background and experience, we will tend to choose one type of explanation over another. My body isn't doing what I want it to do – maybe I have a neurological disease – versus maybe there is some outside force doing it for me.

2. Strawberry Fields Forever

1   David, A.S., 'On the Impossibility of Defining Delusions', *Philosophy, Psychiatry, & Psychology*, 6, 1999, pp. 17–20.

2   If I said that I had captained England in the 1950 World Cup in Brazil, that would be a delusion (specifically a delusional memory) which clearly defied logic since I hadn't been born yet. And I am willing to accept that I might not have made the team.

3   Modern neuropsychology shies away from the strict approach of assigning a problem to one brain region or another, and prefers to describe deficits according to the process in question. Set shifting, or problem solving more generally, is usually classified as an 'executive function'.

4   Noyes, R., Jr. and Kletti, R., 'Depersonalization in the Face of Life-Threatening Danger: An Interpretation', *OMEGA – Journal of Death and Dying*, 7, 1976, pp. 103–14.

5   Ciaunica, A. and Charlton, J. (June 21 2018). *When the Self Slips.* [Online]. (https://aeon.co/essays/what-can-depersonalisation-disorder-say-about-the-self). Aeon. (Accessed 25 June 2018).

6   Sierra, M., Senior, C., Dalton, J., *et al.*, 'Autonomic Response in Depersonalization Disorder', *Archives of General Psychiatry*, 59, 2002, pp. 833–8.

7   Ellis, H.D., Whitley, J. and Luauté, J.P., 'Delusional Misidentification: The Three Original Papers on the Capgras, Frégoli and Inter-metamorphosis Delusions', *History of Psychiatry*, 5, 1994, pp. 117–8.

8   Young, A. and Leafhead, K., 'Betwixt Life and Death: Case Studies of the Cotard Delusion', in *Method in Madness: Case Studies in Cognitive Neuropsychiatry*, eds PW Halligan and JC Marshall (Hove East Sussex: Psychology Press, 1996), pp. 147–71.

9   Ben-Naim, E., Vazques, F. and Redner, S., 'What Is the Most Competitive Sport?', *arXiv:physics*, 0512143 v1, 15 December 2005.

3. Losing My Religion

1   Freud, S., 'Mourning and Melancholia', in *The Standard Edition of the Complete Psychological Works of Sigmund Freud, Volume XIV (1914–1916): On the History of the Psycho-Analytic Movement, Papers on Metapsychology and Other Works*, ed. J. Strachey (New York: Norton, 1976), pp. 237–58.

2   Brown, G.W. and Harris, T., *Social Origins of Depression*. (London: Tavistock, 1978).

3   This is a very comprehensive but technical review of the topic by Mark Williams and colleagues on which I have drawn. See Williams, J.M.G., Barnhofer, T., Crane, C., *et al.*, 'Autobiographical Memory Specificity and Emotional Disorder', *Psychological Bulletin*, 133, 2007, pp. 122–48.

4   Neeleman, J., 'Suicide as a Crime in the UK: Legal History, International Comparisons and Present Implications', *Acta Psychiatrica Scandinavica*, 94, 1996, pp. 252–7.

5   Durkheim, E., *On Suicide*, ed. R. Sennett. Trans. R. Buss, 1897. (London: Penguin Classics, 2006).

6   Dervic, K., Oquendo, M.A., Grunebaum, M.F., *et al.*, 'Religious Affiliation and Suicide Attempt', *American Journal of Psychiatry*, 161, 2004, pp. 2303–8.

7   Thomas, K. and Gunnell, D., 'Suicide in England and Wales 1861–2007: A Time–Trends Analysis', *International Journal of Epidemiology*, 39, 2010, pp. 1464–75.

8   Hawton, K., Bergen, H., Simkin, S., *et al.*, 'Long Term Effect of Reduced Pack Sizes of Paracetamol on Poisoning Deaths and Liver Transplant Activity in England and Wales: Interrupted Time Series Analyses', *British Medical Journal*, 2013, 346:f403.

9   Rubin, D.C. (ed.), *Remembering Our Past: Studies in Autobiographical Memory*. (Cambridge: Cambridge University Press, 1999), pp. 244–67.

10   This is an article which describes the development of new psychological treatment approaches arising out of work on autobiographical memory: Dalgleish, T. and Werner-Seidler, A., 'Disruptions in Autobiographical Memory Processing in Depression and the Emergence of Memory Therapeutics', *Trends in Cognitive Sciences*, 18, 2014, pp. 596–604.

4. Just the Two of Us

1   See Snaith, R.P. and Taylor, C.M., 'Irritability: Definition, Assessment and Associated Factors', *British Journal of Psychiatry*, 147, 1985, pp. 127–36.

2   Angst, J. and Sellaroa, R., 'Historical Perspectives and Natural History of Bipolar Disorder', *Biological Psychiatry*, 48, 2000, pp. 445–7.

3   Crammer, J.L., 'Periodic Psychoses', *British Medical Journal*, 1 (5121), 1959, pp. 545–9.

4   Many of us feel slightly constrained by a rigid twenty-four-hour cycle. Some prefer to rise early (larks) and find they get a lot done in that early part of the day, while others tend to work up to a peak later in the evening (owls). Such 'chronotypes' have been studied in relation to a propensity to bipolar disorder but without any clear association emerging. But it does seem that bipolar disorder is down to some of our most basic biological rhythms spinning out of control.

5   For a useful collection of academic articles on this topic see: Morgan, C., McKenzie, K. and Fearon P. (eds), *Society and Psychosis*. (Cambridge: Cambridge University Press, 2008).

6   Lewis, G., Croft-Jeffreys, C. and David, A., 'Are British Psychiatrists Racist?', *British Journal of Psychiatry*, 157, 1990, pp. 410–15.

7   MacPherson, W., *The Stephen Lawrence Inquiry. Report of an Inquiry.* [Online]. (http://webarchive.nationalarchives.gov.uk/2013081414 2233/http://www.archive.official-documents.co.uk/document/ cm42/4262/4262.htm). United Kingdom: The Stationery Office. (Accessed 1 July 2019).

8   Fanon, F., *Black Skin, White Masks.* Paris: Éditions du Seuil, trans. R. Philcox, 1952. (New York: Grove, 2008).

9   '*Altérations mentales, modifications caractérielles, troubles psychiques et déficit intellectuel dans Thérédo-dégénération spino-cérébelleuse: à propos d'un cas de maladie de Friedreich avec délire de possession*' (med. thesis, 1952, University of Lyon). As cited by Keller, R.C., 'Clinician and Revolutionary: Frantz Fanon, Biography, and the History of Colonial Medicine', *Bulletin of the History of Medicine*, 81, 2007, pp. 823–41. Friedreich's ataxia is a genetically determined neurodegenerative disease leading to gradual but relentlessly worsening unsteadiness, incoordination and dementia.

10   Keller, R.C., 'Clinician and Revolutionary: Frantz Fanon, Biography, and the History of Colonial Medicine', pp. 823–41; Bulhan, H.A., 'Frantz Fanon: The Revolutionary Psychiatrist', *Race and Class*, 21, 1980, pp. 251–71.

11   Fanon, F., *Black Skin, White Masks*, p. 168.

12   Beauclerk, C., *Piano Man: A Life of John Ogdon*. (London: Simon & Schuster, 2014).

13   There is a Gershwin connection to neuropsychiatry. At the age thirty-eight he started having sudden bursts of unpredictable behaviour, complained of smelling burning rubber and forgot his own music during performances. Although initially dismissed by hospital doctors as 'hysterical' (he was in psychoanalysis at the time), it soon became clear that he had an abnormality affecting the temporal lobe: olfactory hallucinations are a classic sign. He died a few weeks later and was found to have a malignant tumour (glioblastoma multiforme in his right temporal lobe).

14   'Just the Two of Us', 1981, by Bill Withers, William Salter and Ralph MacDonald, and recorded by Grover Washington Jr and Bill Withers.

5. You Are What You Eat

1   Ghrelin is short for 'growth hormone releasing peptide' and was discovered long after I left medical school. I like the name because it conjures up images of gremlins, an apt image for those who become cranky when they haven't eaten.

2   Brain tumours pressing on the hypothalamus may lead to either marked anorexia or overeating. The theoretically fascinating but tragic genetic condition of Prader–Willi syndrome is caused by a deletion on chromosome 15. Children with the condition eat voraciously without experiencing satiety. Initial ideas that the condition

might simply be a consequence of increased levels of ghrelin have not been borne out. See Cassidy, S.B., Schwartz, S., Miller, J.L., *et al.*, 'Prader–Willi syndrome', *Genetics in Medicine*, 14, 2012, pp. 10–26.

3   For those interested in digging down into the technical detail, I recommend these review articles: Anderman, M.L. and Lowell, B.B., 'Toward a Wiring Diagram Understanding of Appetite Control', *Neuron*, 95, 2017, pp. 757–8; Ferrario C.R., Labouebe, G., Liu, S., *et al.*, 'Homeostasis Meets Motivation in the Battle to Control Food Intake', *Journal of Neuroscience*, 36, 2016, pp. 11469–81.

4   Gull was a genuinely eminent Victorian, one of Queen Victoria's personal physicians (an honorific). Admirably, he spoke up for women's entry into the medical profession.

5   Bruch, H., 'Perceptual and Conceptual Disturbances in Anorexia Nervosa', *Psychosomatic Medicine*, 24, 1962, pp. 187–94.

6   Orbach, S., *Fat Is a Feminist Issue: The Anti-Diet Guide to Permanent Weight Loss*. (New York: Paddington Press, 1978).

7   Zipfel, S., Giel, K.E., Bulik, C.M., *et al.*, 'Anorexia Nervosa: Aetiology, Assessment, and Treatment', *Lancet Psychiatry*, 2, 2015, pp. 1099–11.

8   Brain tumours or even more rarely strokes, injuries or malformations can very occasionally lead to symptoms of anorexia nervosa or atypical forms of the disorder. The hypothalamus is the most common site, but cases almost indistinguishable from 'classical' anorexia nervosa have been described where the tumour was in the temporal or frontal lobes, more often on the right side, providing evidence against a simple 'problem with appetite' explanation (see Uher, R. and Treasure, J., 'Brain Lesions and Eating Disorders', *Journal of Neurology, Neurosurgery and Psychiatry*, 76, 2005, pp. 852–7).

9   Freud, S., *The Ego and the Id*, Standard Edition, 19, 1923, pp. 1–66.

10 The so-called non-dominant hemisphere, since speech and language, as Freud reminds us, are controlled from the 'dominant' left hemisphere (see also chapter 7).

11 Catani, M.A., 'Little Man of Some Importance', *Brain*, 140, 2017, pp. 3055–61 (beautifully illustrated and contemporary update of Penfield's homunculus).

12 Rozin, P. and Fallon, A.E., 'A Perspective on Disgust', *Psychological Review*, 94, 1987, pp. 23–41.

13 Rozin, P., Haidt, J., McCauley, C., *et al.*, 'Individual Differences in Disgust   Sensitivity: Comparisons   and   Evaluations   of

Paper-and-Pencil Versus Behavioral Measures', *Journal of Research in Personality*, 33, 1999, pp. 330–51.

14 Phillips, M.L., Senior, C., Fahy, T., *et al.*, 'Disgust: The Forgotten Emotion of Psychiatry', *British Journal of Psychiatry*, 172, 1998, pp. 373–5.

15 Dell'Osso, L., Abelli, M., Carpita, B., *et al.*, 'Historical Evolution of the Concept of Anorexia Nervosa and Relationships with Orthorexia Nervosa, Autism, and Obsessive–Compulsive Spectrum', *Neuropsychiatric Disease and Treatment*, 12, 2016, pp. 1651–60.

16 Bell, R.M., *Holy Anorexia*. (Chicago: University of Chicago Press, 1985).

17 Griffin, J. and Berry, E.M., 'A Modern Day Holy Anorexia? Religious Language in Advertising and Anorexia Nervosa in the West', *European Journal of Clinical Nutrition*, 57, 2003, pp. 43–51.

6. Silent Music

1 Monti, M.M., Laureys, S. and Owen, A.M., 'The Vegetative State', *British Medical Journal*, 2010, 341:c3765.

2 Bateman, D.E., 'Neurological Assessment of Coma', *Journal of Neurology Neurosurgery and Psychiatry*, 71 (Suppl I), 2001, pp. (i)13–17.

3 Hume Adams, J., Graham, D.I. and Jennett, B., 'The Neuropathology of the Vegetative State After an Acute Brain Insult', *Brain*, 123, 2000, pp. 1327–38 (study from the home of the 'Glasgow Coma Scale').

4 First Vintage International edn. (New York: Random House, 1998).

5 Monti, *et al.*, 'The Vegetative State', 341:c3765.

6 Owen, A.M., Coleman, M.R., Boly, M., *et al.*, 'Detecting Awareness in the Vegetative State', *Science*, 313, 2006, p. 1402.

7 The eponymous test was devised by Alan Turing (Turing, A.M., 'Computing Machinery and Intelligence', *Mind*, LIX (236), 1950, pp. 433–60, doi.org/10.1093/mind/LIX.236.433). He argued that if a machine or computational device (or witness) was able to answer questions in a way indistinguishable to an interrogator, from that of another human being, the machine could be said to be conscious. While Turing set out the strengths and weaknesses of this proposition in his paper and it has been pored over and largely superseded since then, an imaginary exchange he used as an illustration is worth recalling:

Interrogator: In the first line of your sonnet which reads 'Shall I compare thee to a summer's day', would not 'a spring day' do as well or better?

Witness: It wouldn't scan.

Interrogator: How about 'a winter's day'? That would scan all right.

Witness: Yes, but nobody wants to be compared to a winter's day.

Interrogator: Would you say Mr. Pickwick reminded you of Christmas?

Witness: In a way.

Interrogator: Yet Christmas is a winter's day, and I do not think Mr. Pickwick would mind the comparison.

Witness: I don't think you're serious. By a winter's day one means a typical winter's day, rather than a special one like Christmas.

Most people would judge the witness in this case to be a human being, on the perhaps spurious basis of a shared understanding of cultural and literary references, a rhetorical style of discourse and, last but not least, a sense of humour.

8   Jaspers, T., Hanssen, G.M.J., van der Valk, J.A., *et al.*, 'Pervasive Refusal Syndrome as Part of the Refusal–Withdrawal–Regression Spectrum: Critical Review of the Literature Illustrated by a Case Report', *European Child and Adolescent Psychiatry*, 18, 2009, pp. 645–51. There are a number of variants on the syndrome that occur in particular cultural contexts. For example, there was a wave of cases described in Sweden, known there as *Uppgivenhetssyndrom*, or resignation syndrome (Sallin, K., Lagercrantz, H., Evers, K., *et al.*, 'Resignation Syndrome: Catatonia? Culture-Bound?', *Frontiers in Behavioural Neuroscience*, 2016, 10:7, doi:10.3389/fnbeh.2016. 00007) in the context of often protracted asylum seeking where families were awaiting an adjudication on their rights to remain. This provoked a polarised political response with some claiming that mothers were manipulating their children to behave in this way as a means of emotionally blackmailing the state, while others saw it as the desperate response of traumatised children (see Bodegård, G., 'Comment on the Paper "Pervasive Refusal Syndrome (PRS) 21 Years On: A Reconceptualization and Renaming", by Ken Nunn, Bryan Lask and Isabel Owen', *European Child and Adolescent Psychiatry*, 23, 2014, pp. 179–81). Another possible variant is Hikikomori, first described in Japan a few years after PRS, as mainly affecting young men who withdraw totally from social interaction,

occasionally lashing out when pressed to do so by others, usually parents. Again, polarised views have been proffered to explain the phenomenon – everything from laziness to video games and the internet, to covert child abuse (see Koyama, A., Miyake, Y., Kawakami, N., *et al.*, 'Lifetime Prevalence, Psychiatric Comorbidity and Demographic Correlates of "Hikikomori" in a Community Population in Japan', *Psychiatry Research*, 176, 2010, pp. 69–74).

9   Lask, B., Britten, C., Kroll, L., *et al.*, 'Children with Pervasive Refusal', *Archives of Diseases of Childhood*, 66, 1991, pp. 866–9.

10 Medicine is full of 'exceptions that prove the rule'. One such exception is 'alpha coma', which describes the presence of waveforms in the alpha-frequency band in a comatose patient – but the rhythm seems to come from a different, more anterior part of the scalp and does not disappear when the eyes are opened.

11 Neurophysiologists call this the 'oddball paradigm'.

12 Balconi, M., 'State of Consciousness and ERP (Event-Related Potential) Measures. Diagnostic and Prognostic Value of Electrophysiology for Disorders of Consciousness', *Neuropsychological Trends*, 10, 2011, pp. 43–54.

13 See page 21. " 'Catatonia' is a broad term that encompasses a group of strange motor behaviours…".

14 McFarland and Company, Jefferson, North Carolina, 2012.

15 Freeman, C.P. and Kendell, R.E., 'ECT: 1. Patients' Experiences and Attitudes', *British Journal of Psychiatry*, 137, 1980, pp. 8–16.

16 Rose, D., Wykes, T., Leese, M., *et al.*, 'Patients' Perspectives on Electroconvulsive Therapy: Systematic Review', *British Medical Journal*, 326, 2003, p. 1363.

17 Luty, J., 'Controversial Treatments in Psychiatry', *British Journal of Psychiatry: Advances*, 23, 2017, pp. 169–78.

18 'Electroconvulsive Therapy (ECT): The Clinical Effectiveness and Cost Effectiveness of Electroconvulsive Therapy (ECT) for Depressive Illness, Schizophrenia, Catatonia and Mania', (England: National Institute for Health and Care Excellence, 2003, TA59; modified 2009).

19 The only watertight study is a double-blind randomised controlled design (where neither participant nor researcher knows who is getting the genuine treatment and who is getting a placebo) and where the placebo in this situation is 'sham ECT', that is, having the GA but not getting the shock – and having this done repeatedly for

six or twelve or however many sessions. Plus, there are no rich phar-
maceutical companies ready to increase their fortunes on the back of
proving ECT's efficacy, so the cost of an ideal study (several million
pounds) will fall entirely on a publicly funded health service or
research council.

20 Aviv, R. (2017, March 27). 'Letter from Sweden: The Trauma of Facing
Deportation'. [Online]. (www.newyorker.com/magazine/2017/04/
03/the-trauma-of-facing-deportation). (Accessed 25 June 2019).

7. We Are Family

1 Gelauff, J., Stone, J., Edwards, M., *et al.*, 'The Prognosis of Functional
(Psychogenic) Motor Symptoms: A Systematic Review', *Journal of
Neurology Neurosurgery and Psychiatry*, 85, 2014, pp. 220–6.

2 Estimates of child sexual abuse are fraught with difficulties. Seldom is
there documentary evidence and reports rely on self-disclosure. In a
recent study which compared people with functional neurological
disorders to other general psychiatric patients, we found similar rates
in both, as reported in the hospital records: around 20% (see
O'Connell, N., Nicholson, T., Wessely, S., *et al.*, 'Characteristics of
Patients with Motor Functional Neurological Disorder in a Large
UK Mental Health Service: A Case–Control Study', *Psychological
Medicine*, 2019, pp. 1–10, doi:10.1017/S0033291719000266). Most
researchers in the field would regard these figures as underestimates
of the true prevalence of abuse.

3 This is a study which used an exhaustive search for, and stringent
definition of, stressful life events and showed that they were indeed
found more commonly in the lives of people with conversion
disorder, especially shortly before they developed the condition
(see Nicholson, T.R., Aybek, S., Craig, T., *et al.*, 'Life Events and
Escape in Conversion Disorder', *Psychological Medicine*, 46, 2016,
pp. 2617–26). A very thorough review of all such studies in the
field confirms this [see Ludwig, L., Pasman, J.A., Nicholson, T., *et
al.*, 'Stressful Life Events and Maltreatment in Conversion
(Functional Neurological) Disorder: Systematic Review and
Meta-analysis of Case-Control Studies', *Lancet Psychiatry*, 5, 2018,
pp. 307–20].

4 These terms drawn from the social sciences can be polarising and are
easily misinterpreted but can make a useful contribution to the

biopsychosocial approach. When Talcott Parsons coined the term 'sick role' he was speaking as a sociologist [see Parsons, T., *The Social System*. (London: The Free Press of Glencoe, Collier MacMillan, 1951, pp. 428–73)]. Society, in his view, functioned by assigning roles to people in various circumstances. He was not saying that people were playing a role in the sense of play acting. He argued that being sick brought with it entitlements but required the sick person to try to get well and do what the doctor ordered, the latter sounding somewhat paternalistic to modern ears. Another American sociologist, David Mechanic, elaborated on Parsons' ideas with the concept of illness behaviour in 1961 and subsequently. He wrote: 'Illness behaviour thus involves the manner in which persons monitor their bodies, define and interpret their symptoms, take remedial action, and utilize various sources of help as well as the more formal healthcare system' [see Mechanic, D., 'Illness Behaviour: An Overview', in *Illness Behavior*, eds S. McHugh and T.M. Vallis (Boston: Springer, 1986), pp. 101–109]. Psychiatrist Issy Pilowsky later argued that some 'psychosomatic' conditions could be illuminated through the lens of 'abnormal illness behaviour' (see Pilowsky, I., 'Abnormal Illness Behaviour', *British Journal of Medical Psychology*, 42, 1969, pp. 347–51) when such monitoring and remedial action become all consuming, or alternatively where obvious illness is denied. We can see the origins of these behaviours in everyday life in those who take to their beds at the slightest sniffle while others insist on soldiering on expecting to be acclaimed for their fortitude, spreading flu to their workmates in the process. Finally, the concept of abnormal *doctor* behaviour has belatedly seeped into these discussions. At one pole it refers to things like over-medicalising and over-investigating the least physical and mental symptom with test after test, and at the other, regarding every prospective patient as a would-be confidence trickster and malingerer.

5   This type of tumour starts in brain cells called astrocytes, literally 'star cells', named after their shape.

6   Kutlubaev, M.A., Xu, Y., Hackett, M.L., *et al.*, 'Dual Diagnosis of Epilepsy and Psychogenic Nonepileptic Seizures: Systematic Review and Meta-analysis of Frequency, Correlates, and Outcomes', *Epilepsy & Behavior*, 89, 2018, pp. 70–8. (In this review of dozens of studies and surveys, the authors found that 22% of people who started out with a diagnosis of functional or psychogenic non-epileptic seizures

also had epilepsy while looking at it the other way round; as in Amy, functional seizures occurred in about 12% of people with epilepsy.)

7   Our current understanding of the link between sexual abuse or child-hood trauma and functional seizures is through 'dissociation' rather than nineteenth-century theories of repression and conversion. This is the mental process of separating oneself off, diverting our attention away from the immediate circumstances (detachment) or dividing attention in such a way that certain thoughts are separated from others (compartmentalisation). (For a full explanation see Holmes, E.A., Brown, R.J., Mansell, W., *et al.*, 'Are There Two Qualitatively Distinct Forms of Dissociation? A Review and Some Clinical Implications', *Clinical Psychology Review*, 25, 2005, pp. 1–23.) Many people will describe this happening to them when they were in the midst of the traumatic experience and that it was a way of coping with it – shutting down, even seeming to separate from one's body to the point of observing the situation from outside. This might be a way of dealing with the fear and pain at the time, but it also becomes a pattern that can be triggered later in life when the traumatic events are reawakened. This may also be what happens when some people suffer from depersonalisation – an enduring state of detachment (see chapter 2). It is this dissociated state with compartmentalisation that leads to a lack of control the person has over their actions. The functional seizure may follow the path of the epileptic seizure, either witnessed or personally experienced, like footprints in snow. What was once a useful escape mechanism becomes out of control and a problem in its own right.

8   This is a good example of a functional disorder arising in the context of an impossible dilemma for which the illness provides a means of escape (see Nicholson, T.R., Aybek, S., Craig, T., *et al.*, 'Life Events and Escape in Conversion Disorder', *Psychological Medicine*, 46, 2016, pp. 2617–26).

9   The kind of multidisciplinary team approach to patients like Christopher is described in this paper: McCormack, R., Moriarty, J., Mellers, J.D., *et al.*, 'Specialist Inpatient Treatment for Severe Motor Conversion Disorder: A Retrospective Comparative Study', *Journal of Neurology Neurosurgery and Psychiatry*, 85, 2014, pp. 895–900.

10   This is called 'Hoover's Sign', invented by Charles Franklin Hoover (1865–1927) and published in 1908. Hoover was an American

physician who worked in Cleveland and was famous for his diagnostic acumen.

11 Nielsen, G., Stone, J., Matthews, A., *et al.*, 'Physiotherapy for Functional Motor Disorders: A Consensus Recommendation', *Journal of Neurology Neurosurgery and Psychiatry*, 86, 2015, pp. 1113–19

12 And the same with running being easier than walking. See http://neurosymptoms.org/ produced by Dr Jon Stone, an Edinburgh neurologist. This website is full of useful explanations, advice and examples of effective therapeutic interventions.

13 The language disorder affecting Amy was first described in the 1860s by French surgeon Paul Broca. He was convinced that it was the left side of the brain, not the right, that produced language, and also that expressive language (speech) could be affected without necessarily affecting comprehension, which, as became clear a few years later, critically depends on regions slightly further back in the temporal (and parietal) lobes, also on the left. Broca's patient had a slow-growing tumour which eventually reduced him to saying just one syllable, 'tan', which became his nickname. Detailed MRI scans of his actual preserved brain specimen have been published (see Dronkers, N.F., Plaisant, O., Iba-Zizen, M.T., *et al.*, 'Paul Broca's Historic Cases: High Resolution MR Imaging of the Brains of Leborgne and Lelong', *Brain*, 130, 2007, pp. 1432–41). That specific area affected by the tumour is now known as 'Broca's area'. Sigmund Freud studied language disorders due to brain damage ('aphasias') in that era before turning his attention to hysteria. Freud, the neurologist, was uncomfortable with the idea that something as complex and subtle as language could be localised to a single bump of grey matter; instead, he favoured a network of interconnected regions (see Wallesch, C.-W., 'History of Aphasia: Freud as an Aphasiologist', *Aphasiology*, 18, 2004, pp. 389–99). It may not be coincidental that at the core of his theory of hysteria was the proposition that the people affected were unable to put into words what was troubling them.

14 Whether this was just a placebo effect or, alternatively, some kind of neurophysiological resetting is not clear. Research is underway, led by neuropsychiatrist Tim Nicholson, to examine TMS in functional weakness in a controlled trial comparing sham TMS with the real thing. His current hypothesis is that it is the demonstration of the

possibility of movement (and not just the powerful suggestion conveyed by fancy electronic equipment and white-coated boffins) which is the key ingredient (see Pollak, T.A., Nicholson, T.R., Edwards, M.J., *et al.*, 'A Systematic Review of Transcranial Magnetic Stimulation in the Treatment of Functional (Conversion) Neurological Symptoms. *Journal of Neurology Neurosurgery and Psychiatry*, 85, 2014, pp. 191–7).

Index

Anthony David is Director of the UCL Institute of Mental Health and honorary consultant neuropsychiatrist at the National Hospital, Queen Square. For twenty-eight years he was a consultant psychiatrist at Maudsley Hospital, London, the country's leading psychiatric institution. A Fellow of the Royal College of Physicians, the Royal College of Psychiatrists and the Academy of Medical Sciences, he has published over 600 peer-reviewed articles and is co-editor of the journal *Cognitive Neuropsychiatry* and the book *Lishman's Organic Psychiatry*. He also wrote the introduction to the Penguin Classics edition of R. D. Laing's *The Divided Self*. He lives in London.